NEW DEVELOPMENTS IN MEDICAL RESEARCH

SARCOIDOSIS

CLINICAL MANIFESTATIONS, DIAGNOSTIC METHODS AND MANAGEMENT STRATEGIES

NEW DEVELOPMENTS IN MEDICAL RESEARCH

Additional books in this series can be found on Nova's website under the Series tab.

Additional e-books in this series can be found on Nova's website under the e-book tab.

NEW DEVELOPMENTS IN MEDICAL RESEARCH

SARCOIDOSIS

CLINICAL MANIFESTATIONS, DIAGNOSTIC METHODS AND MANAGEMENT STRATEGIES

DARREN HARPER
EDITOR

NOVA BIOMEDICAL
New York

Library of Congress Cataloging-in-Publication Data

ISBN: 978-1-63482-891-8
Library of Congress Control Number: 2015939744

Published by Nova Science Publishers, Inc. † New York

Contents

Preface

Sarcoidosis is a multisystem granulomatous disease of unknown etiology. It can occur at all ages, with the incidence peaking at 20 to 40 years. This book reviews the epidemiology, etiology, pathology, clinical manifestations, diagnosis and management strategies of sarcoidosis, while highlighting recent studies that have provided new insights into this unique and debilitating disease. The authors also specifically point out the urological manifestations of sarcoidosis to avoid misdiagnoses and to provide early intervention.

Chapter 1 – *Sarcoidosis* is a multisystem granulomatous disease with *noncaseating granulomas* in involved organs. It is more frequent at peaking at 20 to 40 years. The annual incidence varies among geographic regions, race and genetic predisposition. The disease is from 3 to 4 times more common in black people. These patients often have an acute and serious illness. Sarcoidosis appears later in black Americans. The etiology is unknown, but genetic and environmental factors have been associated with it (as micobacterias or exposure to beryllium). Sarcoidosis can incidentally detected due to radiographic test requested for another reason in about half of patients. Lung, skin and eyes are the organs most commonly involved. Bilateral hilar lymphadenopathy are characteritic features and erythema nodosum is the most common cutaneous manifestation. Löfgren´s Syndrome is known as the combination of eythema nodosum, bilateral hilar lymphadenopathy, fever and migratory polyarthritis with spontaneous remission. The diagnosis of sarcoidosis must be established by biopsy from the involved organ, except those with Löfgren´s syndrome. Angiotensin converting enzyme levels are elevated in more half of people with sarcoidosis, but they do not provide the diagnosis. Most patients with sarcoidosis do not require therapy because a high proportion of patients have an asymptomatic or nonprogressive disease.

Chapter 2 – Sarcoidosis is a systemic disease of unknown etiology that is characterized by the presence of non-caseating epithelioid granulomas, usually in multiple organs. Several studies have shown that sarcoidosis might be the result of an exaggerated granulomatous reaction after exposure to unidentified antigens in genetically susceptible individuals. Cardiac involvement may occur and lead to an adverse outcome: the heart mechanics will be affected and causes ventricular failure, and the cardiac electrical system will be disrupted and lead to complete heart block, malignant ventricular tachycardia, and sudden cardiac death. Thus, early diagnosis and treatment of this potentially devastating disease is critically important. However, sensitive and accurate imaging modalities have not been established. Recent studies have demonstrated the promising potential of advanced cardiac imaging including cardiac magnetic resonance imaging and ^{18}F-fluoro-2-deoxyglucose positron emission tomography in the diagnosis and assessment of cardiac sarcoidosis (CS). Pharmacological and nonpharmacological treatment for CS has improved the prognosis of CS, however, there are many issues that remain to be solved in the management of CS. Here, we discuss the clinical manifestations, diagnostic methods and management strategies of CS, while highlighting recent studies that have provided new insights into the unique disease.

Chapter 3 – *Introduction.* Sarcoidosis is multi-system disease of unknown cause which occasionally involves the urinary system. We describe the urological manifestations of sarcoidosis and how the disease may affect the management of multiple urological conditions. *Materials and Methods.* A systematic search of PubMed® was performed using the keyword "Renal Sarcoidosis" and multiple urological terms. We only included articles from the English literature in our review. *Results.* Sarcoidosis is a disease where non-caseating granulomas form in various organs in the body, particularly the lung whereas genitourinary involvement is clinically scarce. It can also cause a decline in renal function or may present as nephrolithiasis. Recognizing the disease and providing appropriate treatment early in its course may prevent further renal decline. *Conclusions.* Sarcoidosis can be a challenging urological disease to diagnose and treat. Urologists should be aware of the urological manifestations of sarcoidosis to avoid misdiagnoses and provide early intervention.

Chapter 4 – Sarcoidosis is a systemic disease of unknown etiology characterized by small well-formed granulomas in one or more organs. This chronic multisystem granulomatous disease is often diagnosed after a finding of hilar and mediastinal adenopathy on a chest radiograph. The diagnosis of sarcoidosis needs a compatible clinical picture, as well as demonstrating noncaseating granulomas (without necrosis) in tissues, while other diseases with these features have to be excluded. In patients with suspected sarcoidosis pathologic specimens for diagnosis of sarcoidosis can be obtained by conventional bronchoscopy with endobronchial and transbronchial lung biopsy, bronchoalveolar lavage, and recently introduced endoscopic ultrasound-guided techniques (endoscopic ultrasound-guided fine-needle aspiration, EUS-FNA, and endoscopic ultrasound-guided transbronchial needle aspiration, EBUS-TBNA) or surgical procedures such as thoracotomy, thoracoscopy, and mediastinoscopy. The diagnostic tools mostly consist of standard TBNA, EUS-FNA and EBUS-FNA. As in histology, the cytologic features of sarcoidosis consist of granulomatous reaction and numerous multinucleated giant cells containing intracytoplasmic inclusions like asteroid bodies (ABs), Schaumann bodies, and/ or calcium oxalate crystals. The sensitivity of these tools in diagnosing sarcoidosis ranges from 60.9% to 100% (median, 86%); specificity ranges from 93% to 100% (median, 100%) and diagnostic accuracy ranges from 73.1% to 95.8% (median, 86.75%). Asteroid bodies (ABs) are commonly described as star-like, spider-, or umbrella-shaped cytoplasmic inclusions in giant cells of granulomas in sarcoidosis and other type granulomas, both of infectious and non-infectious etiology. The pathophysiologic changes that produce ABs, and the nature and significance of these structures seem to be unclear. As early as 1911, intracellular bodies similar in morphology to asteroids were observed in lung, lymph nodes, liver and spleen of autopsy cases before the general recognition of Boek's sarcoid as a disease entity. In the year 1944, the mode of formation of asteroid bodies in giant cells of sarcoid lesions was described but the histochemical reactions failed to give definite information regarding their causation. It took another 25 years, when in ultrastructural studies, the principal materials forming ABs were reported to be either collagen or microtubules, and suggested to be formed by the epithelioid cells themselves or synthesized by distantly located mesenchymal cells and trapped in between epithelioid cells during fusion of epithelioid cells to form giant cells. We have observed that ABs start forming in mononucleated macrophages/epithelioid cells, which may subsequently fuse to form multinucleated giant cells containing one or more ABs. We suggest that the microtubules/tubulins and cytoplasmic membrane forming asteroid bodies in epithelioid histiocytes and MGCs of pulmonary sarcoid lesions, originate from the ingestion of degenerated cilia of bronchial epithelium, which otherwise play a role in the inflammatory process of sarcoidosis including granuloma formation. This hypothesis is based on light microscopic observation of intracytoplasmic material in epithelioid histiocytes having similar tinctorial character as the degenerated cilia in the transbronchial needle aspiration smears, and also cytomorphological evidence to suggest stepwise development of asteroid body from this material.

In: Sarcoidosis
Editor: Darren Harper
ISBN: 978-1-63482-891-8

Chapter 1

Review of Sarcoidosis

Gema Maria Garcia Garcia*[*], *MD
Specialist in internal medicine.
Department of Internal Medicine.
University Hospital Complex in Badajoz (Spain)

Abstract

Sarcoidosis is a multisystem granulomatous disease with *noncaseating granulomas* in involved organs. It is more frequent at peaking at 20 to 40 years [1]. The annual incidence varies among geographic regions, race and genetic predisposition [1]. The disease is from 3 to 4 times more common in black people. These patients often have an acute and serious illness. Sarcoidosis appears later in black Americans [1]. The etiology is unknown, but genetic and environmental factors have been associated with it (as micobacterias or exposure to beryllium) [1]. Sarcoidosis can incidentally detected due to radiographic test requested for another reason in about half of patients. Lung, skin and eyes are the organs most commonly involved. Bilateral hilar lymphadenopathy are characteritic features and erythema nodosum is the most common cutaneous manifestation [2]. Löfgren´s Syndrome is known as the combination of eythema nodosum, bilateral hilar lymphadenopathy, fever and migratory polyarthritis with spontaneous remission. The diagnosis of sarcoidosis must be established by biopsy from the involved organ, except those with

[*] Corresponding author´s email: geminway21@hotmail.com

Löfgren´s syndrome [1]. Angiotensin converting enzyme levels are elevated in more half of people with sarcoidosis, but they do not provide the diagnosis. Most patients with sarcoidosis do not require therapy because a high proportion of patients have an asymptomatic or nonprogressive disease [1-2].

Sarcoidosis

Sarcoidosis is a multisystem granulomatous disease of unknown etiology. Histology presents *noncaseating granulomas* in involved organs. It is initially presented with bilateral hilar lymphadenopathy, pulmonary interstitial infiltrates and/ or involvement in other organs such as the skin or eyes.

Epidemiology

Sarcoidosis can occur at all ages, with the *incidence* peaking at 20 to 40 years [1].

The annual incidence varies among geographic regions, race and genetic predisposition. In countries of northern Europe the annual incidence is high (5-40 cases per 100.000 people) and Japan it is very low (1-2 cases per 100.000 people) [1].

The European *prevalence* is estimated at 40 cases per 100.000 population [2].

This disease is from 3 to 4 times more common in black people. These patients often have an acute and serious illness. Sarcoidosis appears later in black Americans, approximately in the fourth decade of life [1].

Etiology

The etiology is unknown, but genetic and environmental factors have been associated [1]:

- *Environmental factors*: It has been described the relationship of sarcoidosis with occupational and environmental exposure to *beryllium*. A serie of cases suggest that exposure to dust produced in

World Trade Center disaster of New York in 2.001 was associated with an increased incidence of pulmonary sarcoidosis over the next five years.

- *Infectious factors*: Many *microorganisms*, especially *micobacteria*, have been considered as possible etiologic agents of sarcoidosis.
- *Genetic factors*: The first-degree relatives have increased risk for developing sarcoidosis, suggesting the possibility of a genetic contribution. The different clinical manifestations of sarcoidosis have been associated with the antigens of the major histocompatibility complex (MHC). However, the pattern varies by race of the study population, reflecting the clinical heterogeneity of sarcoidosis. Most include HLA-associated *HLA-A1, HLA-B8, HLA-DR3* and *HLA-DR4.* Other genes have been described that may increase that may increase susceptibility to developing sarcoidosis as annexin A11 (ANXA11) [3] or overexpression of genes of metalloproteases (MMP-12) [4] that involved in lung remodeling.
- *Immunologic factors*: Most lymphocytes in granuloma and bronchoalveolar lavage (BAL) are CD4+ T-cells. These cells produce IL-2, INF-γ and other cytokines characteristics of the Th1 phenotype. However, the peripheral blood of patients with pulmonary sarcoidosis shows a T-cell lymphopenia, particularly CD4+ T-cells.
- Several cytokines appear to be important in the formation of granulomas, such as IL-2 that is involved in the proliferation of activated T-cells in early disease. Futhermore, Il-12 and Il-18 stimulate CD4+ lymphocytes to produce IFN-γ. Subsequently, the Th2 cells release cytokines, as IL-4, which stimulate production of extracellular matrix proteins and chemotactic factors that attract fibroblasts and promote the evolution to fibrosis.

Pathology

The main histological feature is the development of noncaseating granulomas [1]. The granulomas are composed of macrophages, epithelioid cells and multinucleated giant cells in the central area, which is encircled by lymphocytes, mainly CD4+ T-cells and even fibrobalsts [1]. The multinucleated giant cells often contain cytoplasmic inclusions, such as *asteroid bodies*, *Schaumann bodies* or *birefringent crystalline* particles [5].

Clinical Manifestations

Sarcoidosis is incidentally detected due to radiographic abnormalities requested for another reason in about half of patients. Systemic symptoms may present such as fatigue, malaise, fever and weight loss [1]. Up to 30% of patients have extrathoracic manifestations of sarcoidosis.

Lofgren´s syndrome is the combination of *erythema nodosum, hilar lymphadenopathy, fever* and *migratory arthritis* with *spontaneous remission.* It is more common in *women* and is strongly associated with the presence of *HLA-DQB1*0201* and *HLA-DQB1*0301* [6].

Pulmonary Manifestations

Pulmonary involvement occurs in 90% of patients with sarcoidosis and is usually presented with cough, dyspnea or chest pain [1]. The "classic" radiological findings are *bilateral hilar lymphadenopathy* followed by *interstitial or alveolar infiltrates* [1]. Pleural *involvement* is rare (less than 5%) and can result in exudative pleural effusion with a predominance of lymphocytes, chylothorax, hemothorax or neumotórax [7]. *Pulmonary hypertension* is a complication that can affect up to 23% of patients with sarcoidosis [1].

Pulmonary involvement is classified into 4 stages according to findings on chest radiography [1]:

- Stage I: characterized by the presence of bilateral hilar lymphadenopathy, which in 50% of cases is the first expression of sarcoidosis.
- Stage II: consists of bilateral hilar lymphadenopathy and reticular infiltrates predominantly in bases.
- Stage III: reticular infiltrates is usually distributed in the upper lung fields and regression of hilar lymph.
- Stage IV: defined by extensive damage including reticular pulmonary infiltrates predominantly upper fields, volume loss, traction bronchiectasis, extensive calcifications, cavitation and/or cysts.

The high resolution computed tomography (HRCT) can show other findings, such as thickening of the bronchial wall, lung nodules, ground glass opacities or fibrosis [1, 8]. The positron emission tomography (PET) may be useful for identifying granulomatous disease. Gallium-67 pulmonary scintigraphy can show alveolar inflammation, although a negative result does not exclude the disease [9].

The pulmonary function test reveal a restrictive pattern with reduced diffusing capacity for carbon monoxide (DLCO), although it is not uncommon that lung function is normal [1]. The bronchoalveolar lavage (BAL) can be use as a complementary measure to support the diagnosis of sarcoidosis, demonstrating a reduction in the number of CD8 T-cells, a elevated amount of CD4+ T-cells and increased CD4 to CD8 ratio [9].

Respiratory Tract Manifestations

Involvement of the upper respiratory tract include larynx, pharynx, nasal and sinuses [8].

Patients may have sinusitis, epistaxis or nasal polyposis [8].

Endobronchial disease occurs in approximately 40% of patients with pulmonary sarcoidosis stage I and 70% of patients with stage II or III [8]. Severe stenosis of the respiratory tract is rare and can be unwieldy.

Cutaneous Manifestations

The skin involvement appears in 25% of patients and is classified as specific and non-specific bases on histopathologic features [2].

The risk of systemic involvement in patients with limited disease to the skin is unknown. *Specific skin lesions* contain noncaseating granulomas and may appear with a variety of morphologies, but most often appear as papules o nodules [2]:

- *Papular sarcoidosis* is presented with multiple papules that may coalesce to form plaques. Predominate in the face, especially eyelids and nasolabial folds.
- *Nodular sarcoidosis*: the nodules may have 1 to 2 cm in diameter, single o multiple, in the dermis or subcutaneous tissue. *Subcutaneous sarcoidosis or Darier-Roussy sarcoidosis* refers to nodular sarcoidosis affecting primarily the subcutaneous tissue, with asymptomatic,

erythematous, violaceosus or hyperpigmented nodules, predominantly in the upper extremities.

- *Maculopapular sacoidosis* consists of slightly raised, red or brown violet macules and papules, predominantly on the face. These lesions may be asymptomatic or pruritic.
- *Plaque sarcoidosis*: Sarcoidosis can present with oval or annular shaped, erythematous or brown indurated plaques, which typically affect the shoulders, arms, back and buttocks.
- *Lupus pernio* is characterized by papules or purple or erythematous indurated nodules, which are mainly distributed in the face, as the alar rim of the nose. The presence of lupus pernio appears to be associated with an increased risk for extracutaneous disease, mainly in the respiratory tract [8]. Lytic and cystic bone lesions, especially in the hands and feet, may underlie affected areas of lupus pernio.
- *Hypopigmented sarcoidosis* affects almost exclusively dark-skinned people. The lesions appear as oval hypopigmented, well demarcated, round or oval plaques. Erythematous papules may appear in the center of the lesion.
- *Atrophic and ulcerative sarcoidosis* is a form of sarcoidosis with depressed plaques that may ulcerate in a minority of patients, particularly black women. Most patients experience other mucocutaneous and systemic manifestations of sarcoidosis.
- There are *rare variants* of sarcoidosis, as *ichthyosiform, erythrodermic* and *verrucous* sarcoidosis.
- *Scar sarcoidosis* is the appearance of sarcoid granulomas in scar tissue of surgical incisions, herpes zoster or venipuncture. *Tattoo sarcoidosis* refers to the development of sarcoid granulomas in tattoos, mainly of red ink.
- *Alopecia* is a rare manifestation. The initial presentation is usually atrophic plaques or erythematous nodules predominantly in the scalp. If the disease progresses, alopecia can lead to permanent. Alopecia usually accompanies other cutaneous manifestations of sarcoidosis, especially in the face.
- Sarcoidosis can produce a wide variety of *nail changes*, such as *thinning, fragility, onycholysis, subungueal hyperkeratosis, splinter hemorrhages*, or *nail dystrophy* which is often accompanied by bone involvement of the phalanges (called *sarcoid datylitis*). Radiographic examination of affected fingers reveals erosions in distal phalanges.

- Sarcoid can affect the *mucous membranes*. *Papules, plaques* or *nodules* can appear in *genitals* [10], and *nodules, ulcers, gingivitis* or *gingival hyperplasia* occur in the *oral cavity* [8].

The nonespecific lesions of sarcoidosis are uncommon except erythema nodosum [2]:

- *Erythema nodosum* (EN) is the most common nonspecific rash of sarcoidosis. It develops in 25% of patients with sarcoidosis. EN is painful erythematous plaques or subcutaneous nodules located predominantly on the anterior tibial regions. It is usually accompanied by systemic manifestations such as arthritis, edema of the lower extremities and fever. EN is self-limited and may appear in Lofgren´syndrome. Histologically, EN is a septal panniculitis.
- Other types of nonspecific lesions are *cutaneous calcinosis*, *erythema multiforme* and *Sweet syndrome*.

Ophthalmologic Manifestations

Ocular involvement occurs in up to 20% of patients with sarcoidosis and is the form of the presentation in 5% of cases [11]. Manifestations include *anterior uveitis, posterior uveitis, retinal vasculitis, keratoconjunctivitis* and *conjunctival follicles*.

The combination of anterior uveitis, hypertrophy of the parotid gland, facial paralysis and fever is known as *Heerfordt´s syndrome* (*uveoparotid fever*) [11].

Sarcoidosis also affects the extraocular tissues, including the extraocular muscles, the optic sheath and especially lacrimal glands, which may present as a *palpable mass* or *orbital inflammation*.

Musculoskeletal Manifestations

Up to 40% of patients with sarcoidosis have musculoskeletal manifestations as arthropathy, bone injury or muscle disease. Approximately on quarter of patients with sarcoidosis have an associated arthropathy [12]:

- *Acute arthritis* can occur alone or as part of *Lofgren´s symdrome.* Arthritis is usually *oligoarticular, symmetrical*, often bilateral and predominantly in the lower extremities. A third of patients develop persistent arthritis, particularly those with high levels of angiotensin converting enzyme (ACE) in the presentation. Joint effusion is usually inflammatory. Tenosynovitis of the Achilles tendon and the flexor tendons of fingers and wrist is common.
- *Chronic arthritis* is usually *oligoarticular* or *polyarticular*, sometimes erosive, in ankles, knees, hands, wrists, metacarpophalangeal and proximal interphalangeal joints. It is often associated with involvement of the lung parenchyma, elevated ACE and *deformities*, as Jaccoud´s type.

Skeletal muscle may be affected by more than half of the patients, but less than 3% have symptoms [12]. The patients can develop insidious proximal muscle weakness similar to *steroid myopathy* or *acute myopathy* with elevated muscle enzymes and less frequently, *painful nodular myopathy.* The *respiratory muscles* may also be affected [12]. *Electromyogram* may reveal a *myopathic* pattern and imaging studies, particularly magnetic resonance, can help distinguish the different types of myopathy and direct the location of a *muscle biopsy* to increase performance [12].

Bone involvement occurs in approximately 5% of patients and it is a chronic and serious disorder. When it is the first manifestation of sarcoidosis, it is usually accompanied by infiltrative skin lesions [12]. Approximately half of affected patients are asymptomatic. *Focal bone lesions* are more common in the proximal and middle phalanges. *Dactylitis* may also be present. Multiple *cystic bone lesions* are typical and are usually detected by radiography, but in some cases can only be seen on magnetic resonance [12]. The involvement of the skull may be associated with lupus pernio and painless nodules of the scalp, nose and malar region. *Sclerotic bone lesions* are uncommon and usually affect the bones of the pelvis, spine and ribs [12]. The MRI is useful in the diagnosis of vertebral sarcoidosis. *Osteopenia and osteoporosis* may be secondary to sarcoidosis or treatment with corticosteroids [10].

Renal Manifestations

Clinically significant renal involvement is an occasional problem in sarcoidosis although histological evidence can reach half the cases.

Hypercalciuria is the most important cause of renal disease. Granulomatous interstitial nephritis, glomerular disease and obstructive uropathy are less frequent [1, 13]:

- Activated pulmonary macrophages produce calcitriol, which increase absorption of dietary calcium leading to *hypercalciuria* and less frequently, *hypercalcemia*. Most patients are asymptomatic, but in some cases can cause *nephrocalcinosis, nephrolithiasis, renal failure* or *polyuria. Nephrocalcinosis* is the most common cause of chronic kidney disease in patients with sarcoidosis.
- *Granulomatous interstitial nephritis* is not uncommon in sarcoidosis. Most affected patients have diffuse active sarcoidosis, although some of them have an isolated elevation of serum creatinine and a few extrarenal manifestations. Urinalysis may be normal or show sterile pyuria or mild proteinuria. Some patients with sarcoidosis develop *acute tubulointerstitial nephritis with uveitis syndrome* (TINU).
- *Glomerular involvement* is rare in sarcoidosis. *Membranous nephropathy, IgA nephropathy, minimal change disease* or *proliferative glomerulonephritis* have been described.
- *Obstructive uropathy* in sarcoidosis may be due to *retroperitoneal lymph node involvement, retroperitoneal fibrosis or ureteral stones.* The retroperitoneal fibrosis may also compromise the renal artery, which can be affected by a *sarcoid vasculitis* and associated with *hypertension.*

Cardiovascular Manifestations

Clinical evidence of myocardial involvement is present in 5% of patients with sarcoidosis, although autopsies indicate that subclinical cardiac involvement is present in 20-30% of cases [14]. Systolic and diastolic heart failure occurs when there is an extensive granulomatous infiltration of the myocardium, which may even develop left ventricular aneurysms [14].

Conduction abnormalities are common, such as supraventricular or ventricular arrhythmias [14]. Heart block is the most common finding in younger patients with clinically evident cardiac sarcoidosis. *Sudden death* due to ventricular tachyarrhythmias or conduction blocks can represent up to 65% of deaths due to cardiac sarcoidosis [14].

Mitral regurgitation is the most frequent *valvular dysfunction* in sarcoidosis [1]. The infiltration of the tricuspid valve and, more rarely, of the aortic valve and root, can cause aortic regurgitation and aneurysm formation.

Granulomatous inflammation localized in coronary arteries can produce electrocardiographic findings and clinical symptoms related to a *myocardial infarction*. Clinical *pericarditis* is rare. Pericardial effusion or a granulomatous mass in the left atrium similar to mixoma may also occur [14].

Endomyocardial biopsy may be useful in patients without other manifestations of sarcoidosis [14]. False negative results may occur due to the patchy distribution of granulomas, so a negative biopsy does not exclude the diagnosis. *Echocardiography* cannot identify microscopic granulomas and cannot exclude the presence of cardiac sarcoidosis. The *single-photon emission computed tomography* (SPECT) can identify myocardial involvement by sarcoidosis and exclude cardiac dysfunction secondary to coronary artery disease. The *cardiac magnetic resonance* and PET may be useful in diagnosis of cardiac sarcoidosis [1].

Nervous System Manifestations

Neurologic complications occur in approximately 5% of patients with sarcoidosis.

They can be the clinical presentation and affect to central or peripheral nervous system [1, 9].

One third of patients with neurosarcoidosis may develop more than one neurologic manifestation. Clinical manifestations are varied and include the following [9]:

- *Peripheral facial paralysis* is the *mononeuropathy cranial* most common and develops up to half of patients with neurosarcoidosis. *Optic neuropathy* and cranial nerve VIII dysfunction may also occur.
- Granulomas with perivascular distribution may produce partial or generalized *seizures*. According to affected anatomical area, patients may have *cognitive or behavioral impairment*, *focal neurologic deficits*. *Hydrocephalus* can also develop [6].
- *Neuroendocrine dysfunction* is due to inflammation of the hypothalamus and / or pituitary, leading to polyuria or disorders in thirst, sleep or temperature. Pituitary or hypothalamic lesions can also cause thyroid, gonadal or adrenal [10].

- *Myelopathy* or *radiculopathy* are due to granulomatous inflammation in the spinal cord.
- *Meningeal involvement* may manifest as an acute aseptic meningitis, chronic meningitis or a meningeal mass.
- *Peripheral neuropathy* can occur as *mononeuropathy*, *mononeuritis multiplex* or *sensorimotor* o *autonomic polyneuropathies*. Electromyography usually reveals an axonal neuropathy. It has also described an acute generalized demyelinating motor polyneuropathy similar to Guillain-Barré syndrome [15]. *Carpal tunnel syndrome* is more common in patients with sarcoidosis than the general population.

The diagnosis of neurosarcoidosis is more difficult if the sarcoidosis is not diagnosed.

Diagnostic tests should be guided by clinical [9]. *Brain magnetic resonance* is the modality of choice, although analysis of *cerebrospinal fluid, electroencephalography, evoked potentials, electromyography or angiography* may be necessary.

Brain, meningeal or spinal cord *biopsy* must be reserved when the diagnosis is not reached or progressive neurologic deterioration occurs despite treatment [9].

Gastrointestinal Manifestations

Gastrointestinal involvement in sarcoidosis is rare, although the subclinical incidence may be much larger [16]:

- *Stomach* is the most frequently affected portion and *abdominal pain* is the predominant symptom. Nausea and vomiting may occur in patients with *pyloric obstruction.*
- Clinically evident *pancreatic sarcoidosis* is rare and the prognosis is good.
- *Liver* is almost always involved in patients with gastrointestinal sarcoidosis, although the clinical expression is variable. Most patients are asymptomatic and have only biochemical changes (usually, elevated alkaline phosphatase and aminotransferases). The ECA level may be elevated. It is uncommon to develop complicatios such as

hepatic vein thrombosis or *portal hypertension.* The diagnosis is suggested by *liver biopsy.*

Other Manifestations

Reticuloendothelial system involvement is common in sarcoidosis. It can manifest as *peripheral lymphadenopathy*, hepatomegaly or *splenomegaly.* Hypersplenism can cause *anemia*, leucopenia and *thrombocytopenia* [17].

The female genital tract involvement is rare. Systemic sarcoidosis does not usually affect fertility and does not increase the incidence of obstetric or fetal complications [10]. Sarcoidosis can affect the testicles, although recurrent epididymitis due to sarcoidosis is rare [10].

Sarcoidosis can affect the *thyroid gland* and cause *diffuse goiter* or rarely a *solitary thyroid nodule.* Almost all patients are *euthyroid*, although *clinical hypothyroidism* is caused by diffuse replacement of thyroid tissue [10].

Involvement of the *exocrine glands* can also be seen in sarcoidosis. *Painful swelling of the salivary glands* occurs in 4% of patients. *Xerostomia* and *keratoconjunctivitis sicca* may also appear, similar to those observed in Sjögren´s syndrome [12].

Diagnosis

There is no definitive test for the diagnosis of sarcoidosis, which requires the presence of compatible clinical and radiological manifestations, exclusion of other diseases that may present similarly, and histopathological detection of noncaseating granulomas [1].

A variety of laboratory abnormalities are frequently observed in patients with sarcoidosis, such as *anemia, elevated erythrocyte sedimentation rate* or *hypergammaglobulinemia. Hypercalciuria* is more common than *hypercalcemia. Angiotensin converting enzyme* (ACE) in serum is elevated in 60% of patients with sarcoidosis. Tissue levels are very high. False positives are rare (less than 10%), but enough to limit their usefulness in the diagnosis and monitoring [1].

Patients with Lofgren´s syndrome do not require biopsy because it is a self-limiting process. The remaining patients required a biopsy to confirm the diagnosis. Biopsies should be made on accessible lesions as palpable lymph nodes or skin lesions [1]. Erythema nodosum biopsy shows no granulomas, otherwise panniculitis, so that there should not be biopsied [1].

Bronchoscopy with transbronchial lung biopsy or biopsy of visible endobronchial lesions is currently the method of choice if there is no easily accessible peripheral lesion. When the diagnosis is not obtained, mediastinal lymph node biopsy via mediastinoscopy or lung biopsy via thoracoscopy or thoracotomy must be performed [1].

Therapy

Treatment of Pulmonary Sarcoidosis

Most patients with pulmonary sarcoidosis do not require treatment because high proportion of them have asymtomatic, nonprogressive disease or spontaneous remission [1].

Oral corticosteroids are the most used drugs for control of symptoms and radiographic abnormalities, although not necessarily spirometry [1, 6]. The side effects of steroids and the uncertain effect of long-term treatment make it important to select patients [1, 6]:

- Therapy with oral corticosteroids is not recommended in *asymptomatic patients* with pulmonary sarcoidosis (generally stage I), unless concomitant extrapulmonary disease itself can justify. For patients with *symptomatic pulmonary sarcoidosis* in stage II or III disease and moderate or severe abnormal lung function, *oral corticosteroids* (prednisone 20-40 mg/day) is recommended for 4-6 weeks.
- *Inhaled corticosteroids* are indicated in patients with cough (with or without airway hyperreactivity), stage I or II radiographic involvement and slight alterations in lung function. *Budesonide* is the most studied agent and can be used as an alternative to long-term low-dose prednisone (5-10 mg daily) in the control of chronic pulmonary sarcoidosis.
- Patients with *acute respiratory failure* or *cardiac*, *neurologic*, *ocular* or *upper airway tract* symptoms may require high doses of oral corticosteroids (80-100 mg / day) for 4-12 weeks.

A maintenance dose of prednisone of 10-20 mg daily is neccesary to prevent worsening of the disease for at least 6-8 months until complete one year of treatament [1]. About one-third of patients have a relapse after reduction or discontinuation of therapy. When the relapse occurs after tapering of the prednisone, the dose must be increased to the last effective dose and maintained for 4-6 months. If there is no improvement after 3 months, prednisona should be increased to the initial effective dose prednisone until reaching improvement (usually 3-6 months) [1].

When patients do not tolerate the side effects of steroids or disease can not be controlled with lower doses of prednisone (10-15 mg/day), it is recommended to rule out other diseases (infectious complications, heart failure, thromboembolic disease or pulmonary hypertension) and begin treatment with immunosuppressive [6]. The agents that have had benefits are *methotrexate*, *azathioprine, leflunomide* and *antimalarial agents* [1, 6]. Tumor necrosis factor antagonist (*anti-TNF) are* reserved for patients with persistent disease despite treatment with corticosteroids and at least one second-line agent (eg, methotrexate) [1, 6].

Several drugs have been proposed for refractory sarcoidosis, such as *cyclophosphamide, mycophenolate mofetil, chlorambucil, cyclosporine, tetracyclines, pentoxifylline* or *thalidomide* [1, 6].

Lung transplantation may be an option for patients with advanced pulmonary fibrosis and associated pulmonary hypertension. Survival rates after lung transplantation are comparable to those of other indications. Sarcoidosis may recur after transplantation, although the incidence is not known [1].

Management of Cutaneous Sarcoidosis

Treatment is not necessary in all patients with cutaneous sarcoidosis due to up to two thirds of cases have spontaneous remission. Treatment should be considered in patients with disfiguring, symptomatic, ulcerating or progressively worsening lesions. The options available include local and systemic treatments [2].

Patients with *localized cutaneous disease* may benefit from local treatments.

It is suggested to start superpotent *topical steroids* (clobetasol propionate 1 or 2 times a day with occlusion) on the trunk or limbs [2]. It is recommended medium-potency agents for the treatment of facial injuries due to the risk for steroid-induced skin atrophy.

An exception is *lupus pernio,* which usually requires the application of *high-potency* and even *intralesional corticosteroid.*

If there is no improvement after one month of treatment, topical corticosteroids should be discontinued and start *intralesional corticosteroids* (triamcinolone acetonide every 3-4 weeks until resolution of the lesion) or *systemic therapy* [2].

Topical steroid therapy can be used as an additional intervention to systemic drug.

When local therapy is ineffective in patients with *extensive skin involvement*, systemic agent must be intiated [2]:

- It is recommended to start with doses of *prednisone* of 20-40 mg per day. If there is no improvement in two weeks, prednisone can be increased to 1 mg/kg/day and initiate simultaneous treatment with *hydroxychloroquine* or *methotrexate* to decreasing the risk of relapse when corticosteroids are tapering.
- *Tetracycline derivatives*, minocycline and doxycycline, are alternative systemic drugs that can improve cutaneous sarcoidosis.

Refractory disease is considered in patients who do not improve with previous treatments and other therapies may be effective, such as *thalidomide*[2], *mycophenolate mofetil* [6], *leflunomide* [6] or *anti-TNF* [6].

- *Topical tacrolimus* can be useful in some patients, as in *tattoo sarcoidosis* [18].
- *Oral isotretinoin*[2], *topical treatment with psoralen plus ultraviolet-A light* (PUVA) and *photodynamic therapy* have been effective in some cases [18].
- *Surgical excision* of skin lesions is not recommended due to the possibility that sarcoidosis appears in surgical scars. However, it is an option to improve the cosmetic appearance in patients with severe disfiguring lesions on the nose [19].

Treatment of Sarcoid Arthropathy, Myopathy and Bone Involvement

Treatment of *acute arthritis* is the administration of *nonsteroidal anti-inflammatory agent* (NSAIDs) [12]. If they are contraindicated or ineffective after 2 weeks, it is recommended to start with *colchicine, hydroxychloroquine* or *prednisone* (10-15 mg/day) [12]. When there is no response to these agents, *methotrexate, azathioprine* or even *inhibitors of TNF-alpha* can be effectives[12]. *Synovectomy* may be indicated in resistant cases [20].

Glucocorticoids can be used to the treatment of symptomatic *myopathy* with similar dose used for inflammatory myopathies [12].

Biphosphonates are recommended for the prevention and treatment of bone loss. *Calcium supplements* and *vitamin D* may be administred, although levels of them should be monitored due to the risk of hypercalcemia [6].

Treatment of Renal Involvement

Corticosteroids are effective in treatment of *granulomatous interstitial nephritis* with doses of prednisone up to 1 mg / kg / day for 6-12 weeks followed by a slow taper [13]. In patients who can not tolerate or do not respond to steroids, alternative therapies may be associated, such as *methotrexate*, *antimalarials*, *azathioprine* or *anti-TNF* [13].

Glomerular involvement in sarcoidosis responds to *steroids* [13].

Obstructive uropathy due to retroperitoneal involvement can improve with corticosteroids, although invasive urologic decompression or hemodialysis may be necessary [13].

Steroids and other drugs as *antimalarials* can improve *calcium metabolism* in sarcoidosis [6]. It is not often that the end-stage renal disease requires transplantation, which is usually due to hypercalcemia nephropathy. The recurrence rate is high but there seems not to be an increased risk of acute rejection [21].

Treatment of Cardiac Sarcoidosis

Therapy of cardiac sarcoidosis includes early initiation of *prednisone* at doses of 60-80 mg daily and gradually reducing to a maintenance dose (10-15 mg/day) over a period of 6-12 months [14]. If the disease is stable or inactive, corticosteroids can be decreased and even suspended. Relapses are common after tapering and should be handled by increasing or reintroduction of prednisone to 60 mg daily. Those patients who do not respond or have many side effects to corticosteroids, alternative agents may be administered with the guidelines for the treatment of refractory pulmonary sarcoidosis. The effect of steroid therapy on ventricular arrhythmias is uncertain and some experts recommend an *implantable cardioverter defibrillator* (ICD) as primary treatment in these patients [14]. A permanent *pacemaker* is indicated for the complete atrioventricular block or other high-grade conduction system disease [1]. *Radiofrequency catheter ablation* may be effective in uncontrolled ventricular tachycardia with antiarrhythmic drugs. *Surgery* may be indicated in mitral insufficiency or ventricular aneurysm [14]. Cardiac transplantation can be considered because the survival rates are high [1].

Treatment of Nervous System Involvement

Steroids are the first-line agents for the therapy of neurosarcoidosis and the dose and duration depend on the type of involvement [6, 9]:

- Patients with *peripheral facial paralysis* or *aseptic meningitis* can be treated with 0.5 mg/kg/day of *prednisone* for 2 weeks. *Myopaty* and *neuropathy* require at least 4 weeks of therapy.
- *Symptomatic hydrocephalus*, a *meningeal* or *parenchymal mass* or *vaculopathy* require higher doses of *prednisone* (1-1.5 mg/kg/day) for 4 weeks.
- *Acute neurologic deterioration* may require *intravenous methylprednisolone* (20 mg/kg/day) for 3 days followed by prednisone (1-1.5 mg/kg/day) for 2-4 weeks.

Prednisone should be decreased gradually after 4 weeks of therapy, especially in severe or chronic patients. *Exacerbations* occur more frequently when the dose of prednisone is closer to 10 mg daily. Patients who do not improve with corticosteroids, who cannot tolerate them or who have a contraindication may be treated with alternative therapies, such as *mycophenolate mofetil, azathioprine, methotrexate, cyclophosphamide, cyclosporine, chlorambucil and infliximab* [6, 9]. These patients respond better if a slow dose of prednisone is also associated (10-20 mg/day). *Hydroxychloroquine, pentoxifylline, thalidomide* or *rituximab* are other immunomodulatory agents that are also used [9]. *Endocrinologic deficiencies* should be corrected [9].

Treatment of Gastrointestinal Sarcoidosis

The start of therapy depends on the activity and extent of disease. Asymptomatic patients usually require no treatment. Symptomatic patients who have a lot of *granuolomatous inflammation on biopsy, severe cholestasis* or *portal hypertension, corticosteroids* are the therapy of choice [16]. Prednisone should be initiated at a dose of 30-40 mg daily for 6-8 weeks with posterior tapering to a maintenance dose of 10-15 mg daily over a period of 6 months. If patients do not respond or cannot tolerate the side effects, *alternative agents* can be used with the guidelines for the treatment of refractory pulmonary sarcoidosis. *Other therapies* as antisecretory may be used to depending on the clinical manifestations.

Prognosis

The overall mortality rate of sarcoidosis is less than 5% [1]. The causes of death in sarcoidosis include progressive pulmonary fibrosis and more rarely, myocardic involvement [1].

References

[1] Iannuzzi MC, Rybicki BA, Teirstein AS. Sarcoidosis. *N. Engl. J. Med.* 2007; 357(21):2153-65.

[2] Lodha S, Sanchez M, Prystowsky S. Sarcoidosis of the skin: a review for the pulmonologist. *Chest* 2009; 136(2):583-596.

[3] Li Y, Pabst S, Kubisch C, Grohé C, Wollnik B. First independent replication study confirms the strong genetic association of ANXA11 with sarcoidosis. *Thorax* 2010; 65(10):939-940.

[4] Crouser ED, Culver DA, Knox KS, Julian MW, Shao G, Abraham S, et al. Gene expression profiling identifies MMP-12 and ADAMDEC1 as potential pathogenic mediators of pulmonary sarcoidosis. *Am. J. Respir. Crit. Care. Med.* 2009; 179(10):929-938.

[5] Myers JL, Tazelaar HD. Challenges in pulmonary fibrosis: 6—Problematic granulomatous lung disease. *Thorax* 2008; 63(1):78-84.
[6] Baughman RP, Costabel U, du Bois RM. Treatment of sarcoidosis. *Clin. Chest Med.* 2008; 29(3):533-548.
[7] Huggins JT, Doelken P, Sahn SA, King L, Judson MA. Pleural effusions in a series of 181 outpatients with sarcoidosis. *Chest* 2006; 129(6):1599-1604.
[8] Polychronopoulos VS, Prakash UB. Airway involvement in sarcoidosis. *Chest* 2009; 36(5):1371-80.
[9] Pawate S, Moses H, Sriram S. Presentations and outcomes of neurosarcoidosis: a study of 54 cases. *QJM* 2009; 102(7):449-460.
[10] Porter N, Beynon HL, Randeva HS. Endocrine and reproductive manifestations of sarcoidosis. *QJM* 2003; 96(8):553-561.
[11] Birnbaum AD, Oh FS, Chakrabarti A, Tessler HH, Goldstein DA. Clinical features and diagnostic evaluation of biopsy-proven ocular sarcoidosis. *Arch. Ophthalmol.* 2011; 129(4):409-413.
[12] Abril A, Cohen MD. Rheumatologic manifestations of sarcoidosis. *Curr. Opin. Rheumatol.* 2004; 16(1):51-55.
[13] Mahévas M, Lescure FX, Boffa JJ, Delastour V, Belenfant X, Chapelon C, et al. Renal sarcoidosis: clinical, laboratory, and histologic presentation and outcome in 47 patients. *Medicine* (Baltimore) 2009; 88(2):98-106.
[14] Kim JS, Judson MA, Donnino R, Gold M, Cooper LT Jr, Prystowsky EN, et al. Cardiac sarcoidosis. *Am. Heart J.* 2009; 157(1):9-21.
[15] Saifee TA, Reilly MM, Ako E, Rugg-Gunn F, Brandner S, Lunn MP, et al. Sarcoidosis presenting as acute inflammatory demyelinating polyradiculoneuropathy. *Muscle Nerve* 2011; 43(2):296-298.
[16] Ebert EC, Kierson M, Hagspiel KD. Gastrointestinal and hepatic manifestations of sarcoidosis. *Am. J. Gastroenterol* 2008; 103(12):3184-92.
[17] Salazar A, Mañá J, Corbella X, Albareda JM, Pujol R. Splenomegaly in sarcoidosis: a report of 16 cases. *Sarcoidosis* 1995; 12(2):131-4.
[18] Gleeson CM, Morar N, Staveley I, Bunker CB. Treatment of cutaneous sarcoid with topical gel psoralen and ultraviolet A. *Br. J. Dermatol.* 2011; 164(4):892-894.
[19] Smith R, Haeney J, Gulraiz Rauf Kh. Improving cosmesis of lupus pernio by excision and forehead flap reconstruction. *Clin. Exp. Dermatol.* 2009; 34(5):e25-7.

[20] Limbird TJ. Arthroscopic synovectomy in sarcoid synovitis. *Arthroscopy* 1993;9(5):599-601.

[21] Aouizerate J, Matignon M, Kamar N, Thervet E, Randoux C, Moulin B, et al. Renal transplantation in patients with sarcoidosis: a French multicenter study. *Clin. J. Am. Soc. Nephrol.* 2010; 5(11):2101-8.

In: Sarcoidosis
Editor: Darren Harper

ISBN: 978-1-63482-891-8

Chapter 2

Cardiac Sarcoidosis: Clinical characteristics, Diagnosis, and Treatment

Makoto Orii*[*]*, MD, and Takashi Akasaka, MD, PhD
Department of Cardiovascular Medicine, Wakayama Medical University, Wakayama, Japan

Abstract

Sarcoidosis is a systemic disease of unknown etiology that is characterized by the presence of non-caseating epithelioid granulomas, usually in multiple organs. Several studies have shown that sarcoidosis might be the result of an exaggerated granulomatous reaction after exposure to unidentified antigens in genetically susceptible individuals. Cardiac involvement may occur and lead to an adverse outcome: the heart mechanics will be affected and causes ventricular failure, and the cardiac electrical system will be disrupted and lead to complete heart block, malignant ventricular tachycardia, and sudden cardiac death. Thus, early diagnosis and treatment of this potentially devastating disease is critically important. However, sensitive and accurate imaging modalities have not

[*] Address for correspondence: Makoto Orii, MD. Department of Cardiovascular Medicine, Wakayama Medical University. 811-1 Kimiidera, Wakayama 641-8510, Japan. Phone: +81-73-441-0621, Fax: +81-73-446-0631; E-mail: kori931@yahoo.co.jp.

been established. Recent studies have demonstrated the promising potential of advanced cardiac imaging including cardiac magnetic resonance imaging and ^{18}F-fluoro-2-deoxyglucose positron emission tomography in the diagnosis and assessment of cardiac sarcoidosis (CS). Pharmacological and nonpharmacological treatment for CS has improved the prognosis of CS, however, there are many issues that remain to be solved in the management of CS. Here, we discuss the clinical manifestations, diagnostic methods and management strategies of CS, while highlighting recent studies that have provided new insights into the unique disease.

1. Introduction

Sarcoidosis was first reported more than 120 years ago. It is a granulomatous inflammatory disease with an unclear etiology that affects multiple organs including the lungs, heart, skin, central nervous system, and eyes [1]. Despite extensive research, the etiology of sarcoidosis has not been elucidated, although most evidence points to an aberrant immune response as the pathogenetic mechanism, which is driven by an unidentified antigen in genetically susceptible individuals. Although multiple candidate etiologic agents including microbial organisms and environmental agents have been identified, the results are inconclusive thus far. While the lungs and the thoracic lymph nodes are most commonly involved, myocardial involvement occurs in 20-30% of patients [2, 3]. Isolated cardiac sarcoidosis (CS) can also present in the absence of clinically evident extra-cardiac involvement, though this is somewhat less common [4]. Although it is not commonly fatal, cardiac involvement may be responsible for more than two-thirds of deaths [5]. Five-year survival rates are highly variable ranging from 60-90% in CS [6]. The clinical diagnosis of CS is therefore critically important to the timely planning of therapeutic strategies.

As with most rare diseases, clinical diagnosis and management for CS relies not on randomized prospective data but on observational studies, limited clinical experiences, and expert opinion. Nonetheless, recent reports have helped to organize a rational approach to these patients and have provided key clinical insights.

Epidemiology

Sarcoidosis is a systemic disease with a prevalence of about 4.7-64 in 100 000 and an incidence of 1.0-35.5 in 100 000 per year. The highest rates are reported in northern European and African-American individuals, particularly in women, and the lower rate is reported in Japan [7, 8]. Differences in prevalence and incidence are linked to age, sex, ethnic origin, and geographical location. The disease can occur in both sexes, with a female to male ration of 1:1.46. Seventy percent of patients are aged 25-45 years, although a second incidence peak occurs in women older than 50 years in Europe and Japan [7, 8]. The clinical expression of sarcoidosis is affected by epidemiological and socioeconomic factors. Elderly-onset sarcoidosis is much more common in women and shows higher rates of change in general health and extrapulmonary manifestations [9]. Cardiac involvement has been reported to be as high as 58% and may be responsible for as many as 85% of deaths of Japanese patients with sarcoidosis [10, 11]. In a recent study revealed that the annual detection rate of CS increased >20-fold during the 25-year period in Finland [12]. Nearly two thirds of patients had clinically isolated CS. With current therapy, the prognosis of CS appears better than generally considered, but patients presenting with heart failure still have poor longterm outcome (The Kaplan–Meier estimates for 1-, 5-, and 10-year transplantation-free cardiac survival were 97%, 90%, and 83%, respectively).

The discrepancies in lifetime prevalence and autopsy data, and the apparent large proportion of cases going undiagnosed, likely reflects both the variable presentation of CS (i.e., many are unheralded or asymptomatic) and the possibility that the initial presentation can be sudden death.

Etiology

The exact etiology of sarcoidosis remains unknown. Many studies suggest that genetic susceptibility and environmental factors contribute to disease development [13-15]. Immunologically, sarcoidosis is an exaggerated immune response to as yet unknown antigens. Data on the clinical heterogeneity of sarcoidosis strongly suggest that the pathogen-associated molecular patterns of microbial antigens can trigger or amplify inflammation. There is no evidence that sarcoidosis is an infectious disease; rather, it is likely to be an exaggerated immune response to the pathogen-associated molecular patterns of killed and partly degraded mycobacteria and propionibacteria [16]. Mycobacteria and propionibacteria persist in macrophage phagosomes because the high lipid contents in their membranes makes them acid-fast, and many of their glycolipoproteins are not very soluble and resist degradation.

Histologic Findings in Sarcoidosis (Granuloma Formation)

The histologic hallmark of sarcoidosis, irrespective of organ involvement, is non-caseating epithelioid granulomas. Granulomas typically consist of a compact central area of macrophages that differentiate into epithelioid cells and then fuse to form multinucleated giant cells surrounded by lymphocytes [17]. These cells become the primary sources for angiotensin-converting enzyme (ACE). There is generally minimal necrosis within sarcoid granulomas, unlike those associated with *Mycobacterium tuberculosis* infection [18]. Granulomas in sarcoidosis are thought to form around and isolate poorly degraded antigens as a means of preventing antigen dissemination and further tissue damage.

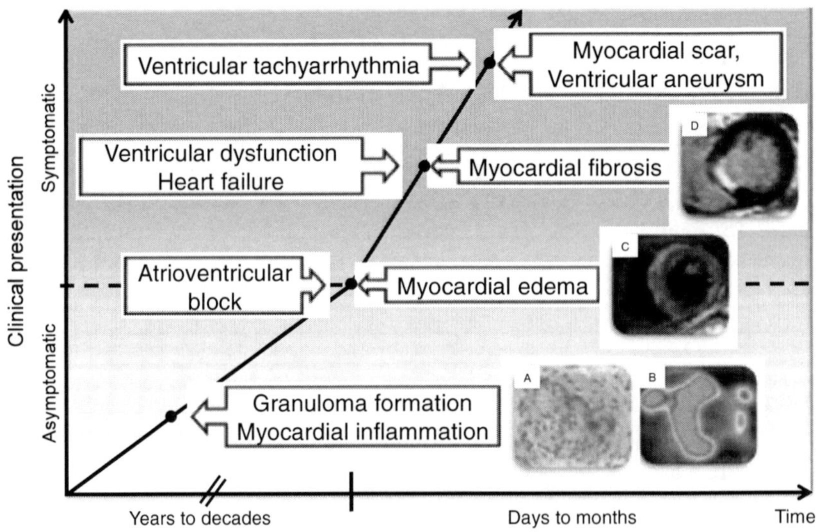

Figure 1. Histopathological stage and clinical presentation.
In this schematic representation of disease progression, the infection point is represented by inflammation, edema, and fibrosis. Granuloma formation (A), ^{18}F-FDG PET of myocardial inflammation (B), cardiac magnetic resonance imaging of myocardial edema (C) and fibrosis (D) are shown. ^{18}F-FDG PET: ^{18}F-fluorodeoxyglucose positron emission tomography.

Why sarcoidosis spontaneously resolves in some patients and progresses in others is still poorly understood. With respect to progressive disease, it has been postulated that the antigen persists, thereby inducing a chronic immune response [19, 20].

Importantly, the detection of granulomas alone is not specific enough to diagnose sarcoidosis, especially non-caseating granulomas that are rarely found by subendomyocardial biopsy in CS [21]. Sarcoidosis is conventionally diagnosed by the appropriate combination of clinical, physiologic, and multimodality imaging. Histological findings of non-caseating granuloma mainly serve to support, not definitively confirm, the diagnosis of sarcoidosis and exclude other potential etiologies from the differential diagnosis.

On the other hand, understanding histopathological stages (i.e., inflammation and edema with the infiltration of leukocytes, non-caseating granuloma formation, and fibrosis leading to post-inflammatory scarring) is important for clinical implications of CS (Figure 1). For instance, ventricular arrhythmias and atrioventricular block (AVB) arising from the earlier inflammatory stage of granuloma formation may potentially be effectively managed with corticosteroids, whereas ventricular arrhythmias arising from formation of scar will likely be ineffective.

2. Clinical Manifestations

The incidence of CS varies by ethnic group, and depends on the type of study performed. An excellent American autopsy series published in 1978 showed that 27% of 84 autopsied patients with a diagnosis of sarcoidosis had CS, two-thirds of whom had clinically significant cardiac disease [22]. Although myocardial fibrosis is nonspecific, it can sometimes be the only manifestation of CS. This series did not consider myocardial fibrosis as evidence of cardiac involvement, so it likely underestimated the true prevalence of CS. In fact, it is becoming more evident that asymptomatic CS is more common than previously thought [23]. In several recent observational studies that screened patients with extra-cardiac sarcoidosis for myocardial enhancement by delayed gadolinium enhancement on cardiac magnetic resonance imaging (MRI), the percent of patients with asymptomatic CS ranged from 19 to 55% [24,25].

CS is most common among older, female Japanese sarcoid patients, with a reported rate of cardiac involvement of almost 80% [2] and the most frequently involved area is the ventricular septum (31.5%), followed by the inferior wall, anterior left ventricle, right ventricle, and lateral left ventricle [26]. Involvement of the ventricular myocardium can lead to left ventricular (LV) and right ventricular (RV) dysfunction and ventricular tachycardia (VT), infiltration of the septum can lead to AVB, and atrial disease can lead to supraventricular arrhythmias, atrial fibrillation, and sinus node dysfunction [6, 27-31] (Figure 1) (Table 1). Although myocardial involvement is most common, sarcoid granulomas can also in rare circumstances involve the pericardium [32] and lead to pericardial effusion and less commonly pericarditis. Patients may present with syncope, heart failure, or sudden death. Because CS often occurs in the absence of apparent disease elsewhere, sarcoidosis should be considered in any nonischemic form of cardiomyopathy, particularly when rhythm disturbances are prominent.

Table 1. Prevalence of cardiac findings in cardiac sarcoidosis

Compete heart block	23-30%
Bundle branch block	12-32%
Supraventricular arrhythmias (Atrial fibrillation, atrial flutter, atrial tachycardia)	23-36%
Ventricular tachycardia	23%
Congestive heart failure	25-75%
Sudden cardiac death	25-65%

Conduction System Disease

Granuloma infiltration can cause injury to the various elements of the cardiac conduction system and result in a variety of conduction disturbances. The severity of block can progress with progression of inflammation and scar (Figure 1). Especially, complete heart block (CHB) is one of the most common finding in patients with clinically evident CS and occurs at a younger age in patients with sarcoidosis than those of other causes [33]. CHB and bundle branch block have been reported in 23-30% and 12-32%, respectively of patients with CS (Table 1). CHB is caused by involvement of the basal septum by granulomas, scar tissue, or involvement of the nodal artery causing ischemia in the conduction system [11]. CS should be included in the evaluation of patients with syncope, especially when it occurs in a younger patient. This was the case in a Japanese study of 89 consecutive patients with no known history of sarcoidosis with high-grade AVB requiring permanent dual chamber pacemaker implantation who prospectively evaluated for CS. Ten cases (11.2%) of CS were diagnosed, most frequently in young women aged 40 to 69 (32%) [34].

Extensive granulomatous lesions in the sinoatrial node subendocardium have been described in previous autopsy series [35, 36], and sinus node dysfunction may also be an under-recognized manifestation of CS [37].

Heart Failure

CS presenting as congestive heart failure with LV systolic dysfunction is a sign that the disease has already progressed to an advanced stage (Figure 1). In a 1976 study observational study, for example, 41% of patients presented with congestive heart failure as the initial manifestation of CS [11]. Progressive heart failure accounts for 25% to 75% of cardiac deaths in patients with CS [6] (Table 1).

In patients with CS, as has been shown in patients with other cardiomyopathies, LV ejection fraction (EF) carries prognostic value. In a review of Japanese patients with CS, 26% of patients were described as NYHA class III or IV, and multivariate analysis showed that LV dimension and deterioration in NYHA functional class were independent predictors of mortality (HR 5.32, 95% CI 1.15-5.84 and HR 7.72, 95% CI 2.33-25.57) [6]. Differentiating CS from idiopathic dilated cardiomyopathy can be difficult. Yazaki et al. retrospectively compared 15 patients having CS and LV systolic dysfunction to 30 patients with idiopathic dilated cardiomyopathy [38]. The CS group had a significantly higher frequency of CHB (67% vs. 0%), right bundle branch block (57% vs. 17%), and abnormal LV wall thickness (73% vs. 17%).

As with LV dysfunction, the presence of RV dysfunction was significantly higher in patients who received appropriate implantable cardioverter-defibrillator (ICD) therapies than those who received no therapies (78% vs. 36%, $p<0.01$) [39].

Atrial Arrhythmias

Supraventricular arrhythmias—in particular, atrial tachycardia (AT) and atrial fibrillation (AF)—are common in CS, with a prevalence ranging from 23-36% in recent study series [40-42] (Figure 2) (Table 1).

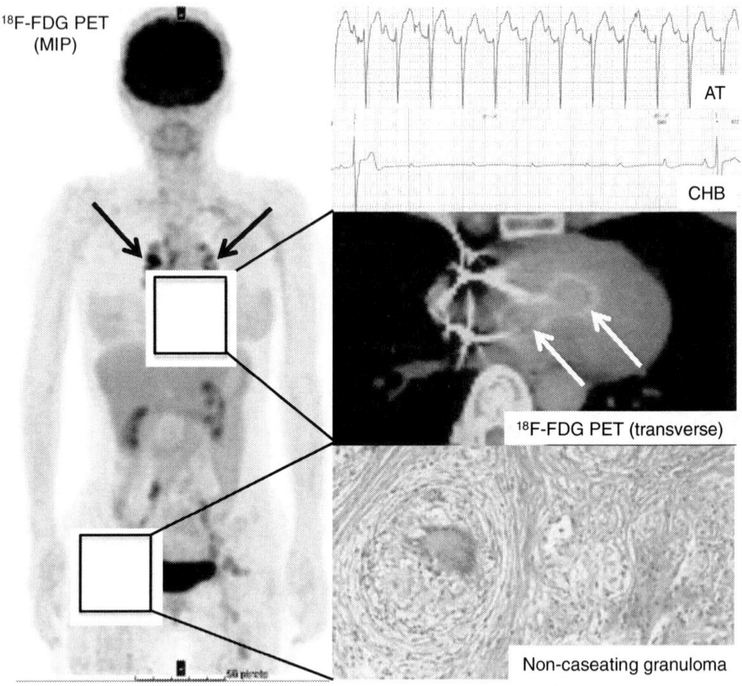

Figure 2. ^{18}F-FDG PET study in a subject with cardiac and extra-cardiac sarcoidosis. A 51-year-old female was admitted to our hospital because of palpitation and syncope. Ambulatory electrocardiogram showed transient atrial tachycardia and complete heart block. ^{18}F-FDG uptake is focally increased in the basal septal wall, consistent with active CS, and is suppressed in other left ventricular walls (white arrows). Whole-body study shows multiple extra-cardiac foci of ^{18}F-FDG uptake in mediastinal lymph nodes (black arrows) and subcutaneous tissue consistent with active extensive systemic sarcoidosis. ^{18}F-FDG PET: ^{18}F-fluorodeoxyglucose positron emission tomography.

A prevalence of atrial arrhythmias was described in a retrospective series, in which 16/44 (36%) patients with evidence of CS by cardiac MRI had documented atrial arrhythmias, the most common of which was AT (18%). In the 26 patients with ICDs in this cohort, 11.5% received inappropriate ICD therapies for atrial arrhythmias [42]. The mechanism of atrial arrhythmias is diverse. In a retrospectively-investigate cohort of 65 patients with CS, a 23% prevalence of supraventricular arrhythmias was observed [40], (9 AF; 3 atrial flutter; 16 AT); these patients went on to electrophysiologic testing to characterize the arrhythmias. The mechanism of atrial arrhythmias was determined to be triggered by activity in 11%, abnormal automaticity in 47%, and reentrant in 42% of the non-AF atrial arrhythmias.

Ventricular Tachyarrhythmias and Sudden Cardiac Death

Involvement of the ventricular myocardium can lead to ventricular arrhythmias by similar triggered, automatic, and macro reentry around granulomas mechanisms [27, 30, 43-45]. Sudden death caused by ventricular tachyarrhythmias or CHB may account for 25-65% of deaths caused by CS, and this may be the initial presentation in 40% of patients with CS [30] (Table 1). Activated macrophages and the inflammatory response associated with granulomatous infiltration in the active phase of CS can play a significant role in the exacerbation of electrical storm in CS patients [39]. New presentations with VT or ventricular fibrillation (VF) should begin with assessment for active sarcoid myocarditis and treatment with immunosuppression [6,45,46]. In other cases of VT in CS, the disease has already progressed to the fibrotic stage and generated scar (Figure 1). As in patients with other cardiomyopathies and VT, scar serves as substrate for reentry by creating both a zone of ventricular arrhythmias in CS patients, when present, can be more difficult to control (both with antiarrhythmic therapy and catheter ablation) than with patients with other cardiomyopathies because ventricular involvement may be more diffuse and heterogeneous. The pattern of scarring that occurs with CS can provide substrate for reentrant circuits involving the endocardium, epicardium, and mid-myocardium.

3. Diagnosis

Japanese Guidelines for the Diagnosis of Cardiac Sarcoidosis

The diagnosis of CS should be considered in two clinical scenarios: (1) in patients with extra-cardiac sarcoidosis, with or without cardiac symptoms, and (2) in patients with no previous histologic diagnosis of sarcoidosis but with unexplained cardiomyopathy, CHB, or VT. Cardiac involvement in sarcoidosis is particularly difficult to diagnose because the manifestations are nonspecific, and the sensitivity and specificity of diagnostic modalities are limited (Table 2). Clinicians must have a high level of suspicion and low threshold to screen patients with sarcoidosis for cardiac involvement, particularly since the initial clinical presentation can be sudden death [10, 47].

Clinical guidelines for the diagnosis of CS were first published by the Japanese Ministry of Health and Welfare (JMHW) in 1993 and they have been used most commonly in the diagnosis of CS and as the reference for comparison of various imaging techniques [48]. Electrophysiological studies should be used to evaluate patients with syncope or significant electrocardiogram (ECG) abnormalities, but their sensitivity and ability to stratify patients by risk are poorly defined (Table 2). A normal electrophysiological study at any one point does not predict future granulomatous infiltration and fibrosis in critical regions. This means that advanced imaging modalities such as cardiac MRI and ^{18}F-fluoro-2-deoxyglucose positron emission tomography (^{18}F-FDG PET) are needed to assess disease activity and management. In 2006, the Joint Committee of the Japan Society of Sarcoidosis and Other Granulomatous Disorders and the Japanese College of Cardiology published a revised version of the guidelines, in which delayed enhancement (DE) in cardiac MRI was added as a minor criterion for the clinical diagnosis [49, 50] (Figure 3).

Table 2. Sensitivities and specificities of imaging modalities for detection of cardiac sarcoidosis

Diagnostic modalities	Sensitivity (%)	Specificity (%)
Electrocardiography	Low	Low
Echocardiography	Low to moderate	Low
^{201}Tl or ^{99m}Tc scintigraphy	Moderate	Moderate
^{67}Ga scintigraphy	Low	High
^{18}F-FDG PET	High	Moderate to high
Cardiac MRI	Moderate to high	High

^{18}F-FDG PET: ^{18}F-fluorodeoxyglucose positron emission tomography, MRI: magnetic resonance imaging.

- ***Major criteria***

a. Advanced atrioventricular block.

b. Basal thinning of the interventricular septum.

c. Positive 67gallium uptake in the heart.

d. Depressed ejection fraction of the left ventricle (50%).

- ***Minor criteria***

a. Abnormal ECG findings: ventricular arrhythmias (ventricular tachycardia, multifocal or frequent PVCs), CRBBB, axis deviation or abnormal Q-wave.

b. Abnormal echocardiography: regional abnormal wall motion or morphological abnormality (ventricular aneurysm, wall thickening).

c. Nuclear medicine: perfusion defect detected by 201thallium or 99mtechnetium myocardial scintigraphy.

d. Gadolinium-enhanced CMR imaging: delayed enhancement of myocardium.

f. Endomyocardial biopsy: interstitial fibrosis or monocyte infiltration over moderate grade.

CMR: cardiac magnetic resonance, CRBBB: complete right bundle branch block, ECG: electrocardiogram, PVC: premature ventricular contraction

1. Two or more of the four major criteria are satisfied.
2. One in two of the major criteria and two or more of the five minor criteria are satisfied.

Figure 3.2. One in two of the major criteria→One in four of the major criteria

Figure 3. Japanese Ministry of Health and Welfare Criteria for Cardiac Sarcoidosis. Delayed enhancement in cardiac magnetic resonance imaging was added as a minor criterion for the clinical diagnosis.

Abnormal cardiac accumulation on ^{18}F-FDG PET was not added to the diagnostic criteria but was included in the additional statements. Several imaging studies have been published on utilizing ^{18}F-FDG PET and cardiac MRI for the diagnosis of CS to date, but almost all of them were validated using JMHW's original guidelines [51-59]. Two recent studies did, however, examine the diagnostic accuracy of ^{18}F-FDG PET based on the revised guidelines [56, 59].

Clinical History, Electrocardiography, and Echocardiography

Patients with extra-cardiac sarcoidosis should undergo a comprehensive cardiac history and physical exam, with special attention to a history of palpitations, presyncope, syncope, or symptoms of heart failure. CS must also be considered in young patients with unexplained AVB, as well as patients with VT and an otherwise unexplained cardiomyopathy.

Kandolin et al. noted that 133 patients developed AVB and became indicated for pacemaker implantation, but the cause of the heart block was not clear in 72 of them. Fourteen of these 72 patients were diagnosed with CS by endomyocardial biopsy. In the absence of signs of extra-cardiac sarcoidosis, 9 of these were diagnosed with isolated CS [4, 28]. Similarly, Nery et al. reported that in the six abnormal ^{18}F-FDG PET scans out of 14 total performed on patients with unexplained monomorphic VT, four patients ultimately were diagnosed with CS [60].

A 12-lead ECG is useful in the screening of asymptomatic patients, given the higher incidence of bundle branch block and QRS complex fragmentation seen in patients with cardiac involvement [61]. Other ECG findings that should prompt further evaluation include frequent atrial or ventricular ectopy, any level of AVB, and pseudo-infarct patterns that may indicate localized myocardial infiltration (Figure 4). Although the ECG is an important part of patient evaluation, it is often non-diagnostic or non-specific (Table 2).

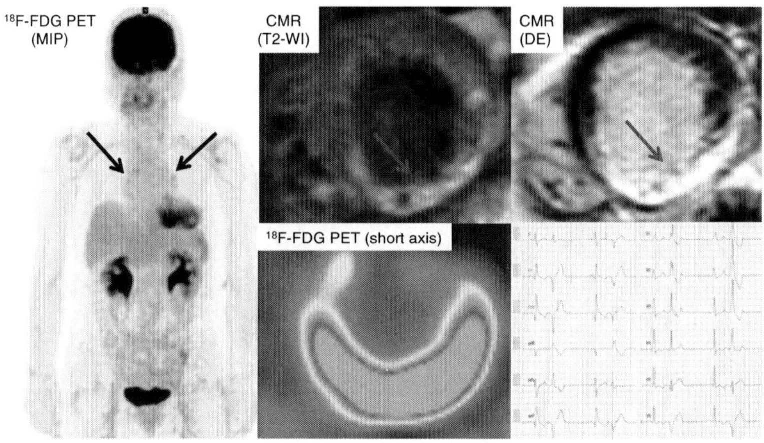

Figure 4. Representative images of cardiac MRI and ^{18}F-FDG PET in a CS patient. Images of ^{18}F-FDG PET and cardiac MRI in a 74-year-old female with pathologically proven CS with frequent premature ventricular contractions. Cardiac MRI shows areas of delayed enhancement and increased T2-weighted signal in the inferior wall of the left ventricle (red arrows). ^{18}F-FDG PET shows focal ^{18}F-FDG uptake in the same region. 3D maximum intensity projection shows ^{18}F-FDG uptake in mediastinal lymph nodes (black arrows). The distribution of the positive finding on ^{18}F-FDG PET image was notably larger than those of cardiac MRI. MRI: magnetic resonance imaging, ^{18}F-FDG PET: ^{18}F-fluorodeoxyglucose positron emission tomography, CS: cardiac sarcoidosis.

Echocardiography is an important tool in the diagnosis and surveillance of patients with CS including abnormal septal thickening or thinning, dilatation, systolic dysfunction, and aneurysm of the LV [62], and consideration of additional testing with signal-averaged ECG [63] and ambulatory telemetric monitoring may also be warranted [64]. However, echocardiography may not detect mild localized myocardial abnormalities which occur in the early stage of cardiac involvement (Table 2). We reported that two-dimensional speckle-tracking echocardiography could identify the myocardial damage detected by DE by cardiac MRI in extra-cardiac sarcoidosis patients who showed no structural and functional abnormalities in heart [23]. This may be a useful method to detect early myocardial involvement in patients with extra-cardiac sarcoidosis.

Histologic Diagnosis and ^{67}Ga Scintigraphy

The only absolute test for organ involvement in sarcoidosis is histologic examination of tissue for the presence of non-caseating granulomas. However, endomyocardial biopsy is limited by sampling and technical errors, and has a low sensitivity of 20–30% [21]. Myocardial involvement can be diagnosed by clinical manifestations and advanced imaging, even in the absence of an endomyocardial biopsy if sarcoidosis has already been demonstrated histologically in another organ, and other causes for the cardiac manifestations have been reasonably excluded. Extra-cardiac biopsies should be performed on the most accessible lesion that appears to be affected with imaging guidance by ^{18}F-FDG PET CT (Figure 2). If no cutaneous lesions or palpable lymph nodes can be identified, then lung or intrathoracic lymph nodes are typically targeted if radiographic and ^{18}F-FDG PET CT abnormalities are detected, due to higher diagnostic yield and lower procedural risk. In cases of isolated CS or negative extra-cardiac biopsy, endomyocardial biopsy may be required to confirm the diagnosis, and yield may be improved with electroanatomical guidance in the electrophysiology lab [65, 66] or with imaging guidance by ^{18}F-FDG PET or cardiac MRI [4].

Historically, radionuclide imaging has also been used in the evaluation of patients in whom CS is suspected. However, ^{67}Ga scintigraphy showed uptake in extra-cardiac sites in 75% of 66 patients with a definitive diagnosis of CS, but in the heart in only 48.5% of them [67] (Table 2). Therefore, radionuclide imaging has been replaced by advanced cardiac imaging including cardiac MRI and ^{18}F-FDG PET, due to the inferior spatial resolution, nonspecific results, and prevalence of imaging artifacts [68].

Advanced Cardiac Imaging

Cardiac MRI

Cardiac MRI has emerged as the gold standard for the diagnosis of cardiac involvement in sarcoidosis owing in part to a lower false positive rate [51] (Table 2). Cine images reveal thinning of the ventricular septum and other parts of the ventricular walls and local heart wall motion abnormalities. Cardiac MRI is superior for evaluation of the heart wall motion, including RV and apex, which is sometimes poorly visualized by echocardiography. Early enhancement of sarcoid granulomas in T2-weighted images suggests the presence of inflammation and edema, whereas DE indicates fibrotic changes and scarring [69,70]. Commonly, the two phases overlap (Figure 4). Smedema et al. evaluated the diagnostic role of cardiac MRI in 58 patients with suspected CS and reported that DE showed favorable sensitivity and specificity of 100% and 78%, respectively [70]. Patel et al. compared the prognostic value of DE in cardiac MRI with JMHW's criteria in an asymptomatic cohort of 81 patients with biopsy-proven extra-cardiac sarcoidosis [71]. CS was detected in 26% of patients by DE on cardiac MRI, but only 12% fulfilled JMHW's criteria. DE was associated with adverse events and cardiac death. These results were confirmed by a more recent study, in which 155 patients with extra-cardiac sarcoidosis underwent cardiac MRI and had a follow-up of approximately 2.6 years [69]. Sarcoid patients without DE, even those with LV dilatation and severely impaired LVEF, did not experience sudden cardiac death (SCD), suggesting cardiac MRI may provide prognostic data beyond that conferred by LVEF alone. In addition to reliably, detecting the disease, DE may also be useful for assessing the response to steroid therapy [72,73]. Unfortunately, however, the test is not effective for patients with non-MRI compatible pacemakers and defibrillators, claustrophobia, or those with renal dysfunction.

^{18}F-FDG PET

^{18}F-FDG PET is a noninvasive molecular imaging technique that is highly sensitive to metabolically active processes. ^{18}F-FDG is taken up by living cells via cell membrane glucose transporters (GLUT) and is phosphorylated intracellularly by a hexokinase into ^{18}F-FDG-6-phosphate (^{18}F-FDG-6-P). ^{18}F-FDG-6-P cannot be metabolized further along the glycolytic pathway and therefore accumulates within cells in direct proportion to their metabolic activity, a phenomenon known as metabolic trapping. In inflammatory cells, especially neutrophils and monocytes/macrophages, cellular activation increases GLUT1 and GLUT3 in the cell membrane and hexokinase over the levels in resting cells [74,75].

Under aerobic conditions, most myocardial energy consumption is derieved from oxidation of free fatty acids, followed by glucose and, to a smaller extent, amino acids. In the myocardium with a low concentration of glucose-6-phosphatase, ^{18}F-FDG-6-P does not enter into further enzymatic pathway and accumulate intracellularly, proportional to the glycolytic rate of the cell.

^{18}F-FDG PET in the Diagnosis of CS

Recent studies have demonstrated the promising potential of ^{18}F-FDG PET in the diagnosis and assessment of CS [51-59,76-78]. Accumulation of ^{18}F-FDG is associated with an active inflammatory process in patients with CS [79,80]. ^{18}F-FDG PET has a markedly higher sensitivity (71-100%) for diagnosing CS in comparison with other radioisotope imaging modalities [53,54,57] (Table 2). Langah et al. also reported favorable sensitivity (85%) and specificity (90%) of ^{18}F-FDG PET CT in patients with suspected CS [55], while a series of case reports have hinted at the promise value of ^{18}F-FDG in detecting cardiac sarcoid lesions [81,82]. For example, Smedema et al. reported that increased ^{18}F-FDG uptake indicated active myocardial inflammation in the heart in a patient with biopsy-proven CS [81]. Similarly, Koiwa et al. demonstrated that ^{18}F-FDG uptake in the heart corresponded well with the pathologically confirmed sarcoid lesions in an autopsy case [82]. Two studies of the diagnostic accuracy of ^{18}F-FDG PET have been published and were based on the JMHW revised guidelines in 2006. Tahara et al. reported that they utilized visual and quantitative analysis using ^{18}F-FDG PET images [56]. Mc Ardle et al. reported the sensitivity and specificity for diagnosing CS as 100% and 83%, respectively, and that CS patients with VT displayed higher cardiac uptake of ^{18}F-FDG when compared with those with advanced AVB [76]. The specificity of ^{18}F-FDG in the detection of CS varies and is relatively low (39-97%) compared with its sensitivity (Table 2). Possible explanations for this include nonspecific myocardial uptake of ^{18}F-FDG in the normal heart [83,84] and early-stage sarcoid lesions in the heart of patients who do not meet the diagnostic criteria for CS [85]. Cardiac assessment can be combined with whole-body imaging to determine the presence and activity of extra-cardiac lesions (Figure 2,4).

Minimizing Physiological ^{18}F-FDG Uptake in the Normal Myocardium

The identification of sites of inflammation is related to the glycolytic activity of the cells involved in the inflammatory response. It is important to determine whether ^{18}F-FDG uptake in inflammatory lesions can be distinguished from physiological ^{18}F-FDG uptake in the myocardium. Although there is currently no consensus on the best protocol for suppressing cardiac ^{18}F-FDG uptake, a recently proposed protocol that combines prolonged fasting [86], dietary modifications [87,88], and unfractionated heparin load before imaging [54] appears to be an attractive solution.

Analysis of ^{18}F-FDG PET Image (Semiquantitative and Quantitative Analysis)

Focal myocardial ^{18}F-FDG uptake has been considered a finding suggestive of active CS lesions. Ishimaru et al. and Ohira et al. visually classified ^{18}F-FDG PET uptake into four patterns—"none," "diffuse," "focal," and "focal on diffuse."—where the latter two patterns were considered to be indicative of CS [51, 54]. Similarly, Langah et al. defined the patterns of ^{18}F-FDG uptake in the heart as "diffuse" or "focal" [55].

In quantitative analysis, the standardized uptake value (SUV) is commonly used as an index of tracer uptake in tumor imaging. The SUV can be obtained using the following equation. SUV= (decay-corrected radiotracer concentration, mCi/ml)/(mCi of tracer injected dose into the patient)(body weight). In CS, a high SUV in the ^{18}F-FDG uptake site has been reported, consistent with visual determination of the site [53]. Okumura et al. divided the left ventricular cardiac muscle into 13 segments. Patients with CS showed a higher myocardial SUV than did healthy subjects. The diagnostic capability based on the above criterion had a sensitivity of 100% and specificity of 91% [53]. Tahara et al. reported that they utilized visual analysis using ^{18}F-FDG PET images, and the sensitivity and specificity for diagnosing CS were 100% and 46%, respectively, but after the quantitative analysis utilizing the coefficient of variation of SUV for segmental ^{18}F-FDG uptake, they achieved a specificity of 97% [56]. As for the use of SUV in the diagnosis of CS, problems that remain to be solved included unstandardized SUV calculation software and differences in measurement values depending on imaging equipment and imaging conditions.

Assessment of Disease Activity during Corticosteroid Treatment

The metabolic signal of inflammation is a marker of disease activity and can be used to guide the need for and response to corticosteroid therapies [56, 57, 78, 89].

Among the case reports in the literature, Takeda et al. reported a case of CS with CHB that had markedly increased ^{18}F-FDG uptake in the basal interventricular septum. After corticosteroid therapy, myocardial ^{18}F-FDG uptake disappeared and the CHB became a first-degree AVB [78]. Similarly, Tadamura et al. documented a case of reduced regional ^{18}F-FDG uptake in the heart after corticosteroid therapy. In their case, myocardial ^{18}F-FDG uptake decreased, as did the serum level of ACE [89]. After steroid therapy, a small study in 17 biopsy-proven CS patients showed a significant decrease in ^{18}F-FDG uptake, while perfusion defects remained stable [57]. Three patients showed improvement on ECG as well. Pandya et al. reported that the recurrence of symptomatic VT was predicted by increased ^{18}F-FDG uptake during corticosteroid tapering [90]. In a recent prospective study of 28 patients with biopsy-proven CS, ^{18}F-FDG PET CT influenced clinical management in 63% [86]. These reports suggest the practical role of ^{18}F-FDG PET in monitoring the disease activity of CS during corticosteroid therapy; however, there are pitfalls in this. First, steroids often induce glucose intolerance along with gluconeogenesis and insulin resistance. Serum glucose and insulin levels elevated by steroid therapy could affect ^{18}F-FDG uptake in target organs including the heart [91,92]. This may preclude an accurate assessment of the effects of corticosteroid using ^{18}F-FDG PET. Also, ^{18}F-FDG PET has a limited ability in showing fibrous regions, although corticosteroid therapy may facilitate the transition from active inflammatory changes to the fibrotic stage. Fibrous lesions can be a focus of reentrant VT. Therefore, decreased ^{18}F-FDG uptake in the heart should not necessarily be interpreted as a favorable finding.

Biomarkers of CS

There are several parameters that can be used to monitor the inflammation of systemic sarcoidosis, including serum ACE, lysozyme, and soluble IL-2 receptor [93-95]. However, in a large-scale clinical study involving 516 patients, Shijubo et al. found that the sensitivities of ACE, lysozyme, and serum IgG were low, at 49.8, 51.7, and 13.8%, respectively [96]. Similarly, no biomarkers with high sensitivity or specificity are known in CS. Japanese data indicate that only 21.8% patients with CS show positive value of serum ACE [67]. Moreover, serum levels of ACE soon return to the normal range after corticosteroid therapy even when disease activity remains high [97]. ACE inhibitors are often used to treat heart failure in CS, and serum ACE levels are therefore likely to be influenced by this treatment. Although the usefulness of the soluble IL-2 receptor has been reported [96,98], no sufficient data have been accumulated in patients with CS. Recently, high-sensitivity troponin T plasma natriuretic levels have been reported to be elevated in CS patients [99, 100]. Determination of atrial and brain natriuretic peptide levels is shown to be useful for identifying cardiac involvement of systemic sarcoidosis patients. We reported that specific monocyte subsets could serve as surrogate markers of disease activity in CS evaluated by ^{18}F-FDG PET [101]. Further clinical investigation is required to develop more accurate diagnostic biomarkers.

Comparing Cardiac MRI and ^{18}F-FDG PET

^{18}F-FDG PET detects active CS lesions, whereas DE in cardiac MRI primarily detects more advanced fibrotic lesions [51,54]. Commonly, the two phases overlap, so the mild to moderate correlation between DE in cardiac MRI and ^{18}F-FDG PET is not surprising [51] (Figure 4). Several studies compared DE in cardiac MRI with ^{18}F-FDG uptake in PET. In a report by Mehta et al., ^{18}F-FDG showed positive findings in 86% of 22 patients with suspected CS, whereas DE in cardiac MRI showed them in only 36% of patients [25]. Ohira et al. similarly reported that ^{18}F-FDG PET (87.5%) was more sensitive than DE in cardiac MRI (75%) [51]. In their study, however, the specificity of ^{18}F-FDG PET (39%) was obviously lower than that of DE in cardiac MRI (88%). When DE in cardiac MRI and ^{18}F-FDG PET were compared against JMHW's criteria, DE in cardiac MRI had a higher specificity but a lower sensitivity [25, 51, 102] (Table 2).

Cardiac MRI has greater spatial and temporal resolution compared with ^{18}F-FDG PET without radiation exposure. It also allows for anatomical and hemodynamic assessment of cardiac function. However, cardiac MRI is not feasible in patients with implantable devices in the heart, which are often used for CS.

The advantages of ^{18}F-FDG PET include the biologic nature of the imaging signal, the potential for identifying cardiac and extra-cardiac sarcoidosis involvement [59] (Figure 2,4), and the feasibility of imaging in patients with implantable cardiac devices. Another advantage for therapy or risk stratification may be quantification. McArdle et al. found higher quantitative ^{18}F-FDG uptake in CS patients with VT than in those with AVB and asymptomatic controls [59]. Similarly, Blankstein et al. concluded after examining a group of 125 patients that abnormal cardiac PET findings, but not JMHW criteria or the EF, are associated with a higher risk of death or VT, indicating ^{18}F-FDG PET offers prognostic value beyond EF alone [52]. The disadvantages of ^{18}F-FDG PET include radiation exposure, false-positive result of cardiac uptake, and the inability to detect smaller regions of myocardial damage. Also, a potential source of error in patients with an implantable cardiac device may be hot-spot artifacts at the lead insertion site on attenuation-corrected images. Although some studies have suggested a significant overestimation of SUV [103], others have suggested that images in the presence of metallic leads can be interpreted without correction for metal artifacts [104]. Evaluation of images without attenuation may be used as an adjunct in cases of suspected lead insertion artifacts.

Electrophysiologic Testing

Electroanatomical mapping, or "voltage-mapping," of the RV can help identify areas of scar, which can suggest the presence of myocardial involvement in patients with extra-cardiac sarcoidosis and no other clear explanation for cardiomyopathy.

Programmed electrical stimulation (PES) can also investigate for the inducibility of sustained monomorphic VT as a means of risk stratification of SCD in patients with CS. One study of 76 patients with CS undergoing PES showed that six of eight patients (75%) with inducible VT went on to have ventricular arrhythmias and ICD therapies over a mean follow-up of 5.6 years, compared to one patient with SCD amongst the 68 patients (1.5%) who had been noninducible by PES [105]. In another study of 32 patients with CS, four of six patients (67%) with inducible VT went on to have appropriate ICD therapies while two of 20 patients (10%) who were noninducible went on to have ventricular arrhythmias or SCD [106]. While these studies suggest a potential role for electrophysiologic testing for risk stratification, these data need to be replicated in larger cohorts.

4. Management

Immunosuppression

Corticosteroids are the first-line agents for the treatment of CS. Steroid-sparing immunosuppressive therapies, such as infliximab, methotrexate, azathioprine, and others are also frequently utilized as well with reports of success [107, 108]. Corticosteroids can eliminate sarcoid granulomas in the heart but that their replacement is by dense fibrous tissue [109]. Therefore, corticosteroid therapy should be initiated early, before advanced clinical manifestations develop [110]. Although data exist showing that steroids improve their prognosis [111], only a few reports have been published and no randomized controlled trial has been done [112]. Yazaki et al. found that 75 CS patients treated with steroids had a significantly better 5-year survival compared to untreated patients (75% vs. 10%) [6]. On the other hand, Chiu et al. found that the benefit of steroids was limited to those whose EF had not already declined <30% [111]. In addition to improving survival, other observational studies have suggested that steroid therapy may decrease arrhythmic burden [6, 45, 46] and even reverse high-grade AVB [27, 78, 112-114]. However, there is no evidence for doses of corticosteroids being appropriate for disease stages. The guidelines for CS recommend a prednisolone of 30 mg/day, but this dose has been used only empirically [112]. We usually treat patients for 4 weeks, and then gradually taper the dose. Maintenance dose of 5 to 10 mg of prednisolone is given for a prolonged period time. No studies have reported on the rate of steroid dose reduction, maintenance dose, or duration of steroid treatment. In particular, since no indicators for the activity of cardiac lesions have been established, the treatment of CS requires further studies.

Antiarrhythmic Management (Drugs, Catheter Ablation, and Indications and Outcomes of Implantable Cardiac Defibrillator Therapy)

Corticosteroids alone can be ineffective at preventing monomorphic VT [27, 43, 45] and some atrial arrhythmias, as disease progression through the inflammatory stage has already led to scar, which serves as arrhythmic substrate and may not be reversed with immunosuppression. Medical therapy alone is commonly ineffective at complete arrhythmia suppression [43], in which case catheter ablation may be indicated. While further studies are needed to determine the efficacy of catheter ablation in CS, particularly in the acute inflammatory phase in active CS, there have been a few published descriptions of experience with catheter ablation for VT in CS. Ultimately, a combination of immunosuppression, antiarrhythmic therapy, and catheter ablation may be required for arrhythmia control in CS.

Betensky et al. reviewed 45 patients (64% primary prevention, 2.6 year mean follow-up period), and found a high annualized appropriate therapy (shock and/or ATP) rate of 14.5% [115]. Predictors of appropriate therapies included lower LVEF and CHB, signifying more advanced disease. Schuller et al. reported on 112 patients (74% primary prevention, 2.8 year mean follow-up period) and found a similarly high annualized therapy rate of 13.2% and an inappropriate ICD firing occurred in 12%. In this cohort, no primary prevention patient with normal LV and RV function received an appropriate therapy, though there were many patients with only mild systolic dysfunction who received shocks and ATP [39]. The rates of appropriate therapies in these studies are notably higher than that observed in large primary prevention ICD trials such as SCD in Heart Failure Trial (SCD-HeFT), where the incidence was approximately 5% per year [116]. The ACC/AHA/HRS 2008 guidelines have a class IIA recommendation (level of evidence C) for ICD therapy in sarcoidosis patients with evidence of myocardial involvement, regardless of symptoms or presentation [117]. The Expert Consensus writing group aimed to further stratify CS patients based on risk for sudden death. In accordance with existing guidelines, secondary prevention ICD implantation is recommended in CS patients with spontaneous sustained ventricular arrhythmias, including prior cardiac arrest (class I). Primary prevention patients with LVEF≦ 35% despite optimal medical therapy and a trial of immunosuppression, if indicated, should also receive an ICD (class I). ICD implantation can be useful regardless of LVEF in CS patients with: (1) an indication for permanent pacemaker implantation, (2) unexplained syncope or near syncope, likely to be arrhythmic in nature, and (3) inducible sustained ventricular arrhythmias (>30 seconds) or clinically relevant VF (class IIA) [118]. Recently, Takaya et al. reported that patients with high-degree AVB as an initial manifestation of CS have a high rate of fatal cardiac events, similar to those with VT and/or heart failure [119]. They concluded that an indication for an ICD, but not a pacemaker system, could be considered in patients with CS manifested by high-degree AVB. For patients with LVEF 36–49% and/or RV ejection fraction < 40% despite optimal medical therapy and a trial of immunosuppression if indicated, an ICD may be considered (class IIB). ICD implantation is not recommended in patients with no history of syncope, normal LV and RV function, no DE on CMR, a negative electrophysiologic study, and no indication for permanent pacing (class III). This patient group is felt to be low risk for sudden death, but should be monitored closely for deterioration in ventricular function or development of symptoms. Finally, ICD implantation is not recommended in CS patients with incessant ventricular arrhythmias or New York Heart Association class IV heart failure.

Heart Failure Management and Advanced Heart Failure Therapies

When systolic function and heart failure do occur, management is similar to other forms of dilated cardiomyopathy. ACE inhibitors, aldosterone antagonists, diuretics, and beta-blockers are mainstays of therapy, in addition to a background of immunosuppression. Cardiac resynchronization therapy may also be indicated in cases of high-grade AVB or in patients with a LBBB and a wide QRS complex.

It has been reported that heart transplantation is also performed in patients with CS, and the prognosis of the recipients is reasonable [120]. Some patients are not diagnosed with CS until pathological examination after heart transplantation or LV assist device surgery. No consensus has been reached on the indications of heart transplantation for patients with CS, a systemic disease.

At least at present, when the supply of donor hearts is insufficient, the diagnosis of CS in patients with severe heart failure is very important, making it essential to initiate immunosuppressive therapy before the determination of the indication of heart transplantation. It was reported that CS apparently secondary to its extra-cardiac counterpart recurred in the transplanted heart of some patients [121], while isolated CS did not recur after orthotopic heart transplant [122]. One-year post-transplant survival has been reported to be similar for CS patients (n=65) as patients receiving transplantation for all other diagnoses (87.7% vs. 84.5%). Furthermore, estimated post-transplant survival at five years was a favorable 80% for patients with CS [123].

Conclusion

The manifestations of CS are highly variable; myocardial involvement can be subclinical, or it may lead to AVB, heart failure, atrial and ventricular arrhythmias, or SCD. Although early diagnosis by multimodality imaging and adequate immunosuppression or nonpharmacological therapy has improved the prognosis of CS, there are many issues that remain to be solved. In the future, multicenter and interdisciplinary research projects will be needed for the achievement of better prognosis of CS patients.

Conflict of interest: The authors declare that there is no conflict of interests regarding the publication of this paper.

References

[1] Joint Statement of the American Thoracic Society (ATS), the European Respiratory Society (ERS) and the World Association of Sarcoidosis and Other Granulomatous Disorders (WASOG) adopted by the ATS Board of Directors and by the ERS Executive Committee, February 1999. *Am J Respir Crit Care Med.* 1999;160:736-55.

[2] Chapelon-Abric C, de Zuttere D, et al. Cardiac sarcoidosis: a retrospective study of 41 cases. *Medicine (Baltimore).* 2004;83:315-34.

[3] Kim JS, Judson MA, et al. Cardiac sarcoidosis. *Am Heart J.* 2009;157:9-21.

[4] Kandolin R, Lehtonen J, et al. Diagnosing isolated cardiac sarcoidosis. *J Intern Med.* 2011;270:461-8.

[5] Roberts WC, McAllister HA Jr., et al. Sarcoidosis of the heart: a clinico-pathological study of 35 necropsy patients (group 1) and review of 78 previously described necropsy patients (group II). *Am J Med.* 1977;63:86-108.

[6] Yazaki Y, Isobe M, et al. Central Japan Heart Study Group. Prognostic determinants of long-term survival in Japanese patients with cardiac sarcoidosis treated with prednisone. *Am J Cardiol.* 2001;88:1006-10.

[7] Hillerdal G, Nou E, et al. Sarcoidosis: epidemiology and prognosis. A 15-year European study. *Am Rev Respir Dis.* 1984;130:29-32.

[8] Morimoto T, Azuma A, et al. Epidemiology of sarcoidosis in Japan. *Eur Respir J.* 2008;31:372-9.

[9] Varron L, Cottin V, et al. Late-onset sarcoidosis: a comparative study. *Medicine (Baltimore).* 2012;91:137-43.

[10] Tachibana T, Iwai K, et al. Study on cause of death in the patients with sarcoidosis in Japan. *Sarcoidosis Sigilim SRL.* 1992;9:307–7.

[11] Matsui Y, Iwai K, et al. Clinicopathological study of fatal myocardial sarcoidosis. *Ann N Y Acad Sci.* 1976;278:455–69.

[12] Kandolin R, Lehtonen J, et al. Cardiac sarcoidosis: epidemiology, characteristics, and outcome over 25 years in a nationwide study. *Circulation.* 2015;131:624-32.

[13] Baughman RP, Lower EE, et al. Sarcoidosis. *Lancet.* 2003;361:1111-8.

[14] Newman LS, Rose CS, et al; ACCESS Research Group. A case control etiologic study of sarcoidosis: environmental and occupational risk factors. *Am J Respir Crit Care Med.* 2004;170:1324-30.

[15] Müller-Quernheim J, et al. Genetics of sarcoidosis. *Clin Chest Med.* 2008;29:391-414.

[16] Negi M, Takemura T, et al. Localization of Propionibacterium acnes in granulomas supports a possible etiologic link between sarcoidosis and the bacterium. *Mod Pathol.* 2012;25:1284-97.

[17] Iannuzzi MC, Rybicki BA, et al. Sarcoidosis. *N Engl J Med.* 2007;357:2153-65.

[18] Rosen Y. Pathology of sarcoidosis. *Semin Respir Crit Care Med.* 2007;28:36-52.

[19] Zissel G, Prasse A, et al. Immunologic response of sarcoidosis. *Semin Respir Crit Care Med.* 2010;31:390-403.

[20] Chen ES, Song Z, et al. Serum amyloid A regulates granulomatous inflammation in sarcoidosis through Toll-like receptor-2. *Am J Respir Crit Care Med.* 2010;181:360-73.

[21] Uemura A, Morimoto S, et al. Histologic diagnostic rate of cardiac sarcoidosis: evaluation of endomyocardial biopsies. *Am Heart J.* 1999;138:299-302.

[22] Silverman KJ, Hutchins GM, et al. Cardiac sarcoid: a clinicopathologic study of 84 unselected patients with systemic sarcoidosis. *Circulation.* 1978;58:1204-11.

[23] Orii M, Hirata K, et al. Myocardial damage detected by two-dimensional speckle-tracking echocardiography in patients with extra-cardiac sarcoidosis: comparison with magnetic resonance imaging. *J Am Soc Echocardiogr.* in press.

[24] Nagai T, Kohsaka S, et al. Incidence and prognostic significance of myocardial late gadolinium enhancement in patients with sarcoidosis without cardiac manifestation. *Chest.* 2014;146:1064-72.

[25] Mehta D, Lubitz SA, et al. Cardiac involvement in patients with sarcoidosis: diagnostic and prognostic value of outpatient testing. *Chest.* 2008;133:1426-35.

[26] Tavora F, Cresswell N, et al. Comparison of necropsy findings in patients with sarcoidosis dying suddenly from cardiac sarcoidosis versus dying suddenly from other causes. *Am J Cardiol.* 2009;104:571-7.

[27] Banba K, Kusano KF, et al. Relationship between arrhythmogenesis and disease activity in cardiac sarcoidosis. *Heart Rhythm.* 2007;4:1292-99.

[28] Kandolin R, Lehtonen J, et al. Cardiac sarcoidosis and giant cell myocarditis as causes of atrioventricular block in young and middle-aged adults. *Circ Arrhythm Electrophysiol.* 2011;4:303-9.

[29] Youssef G, Beanlands RS, et al. Cardiac sarcoidosis: applications of imaging in diagnosis and directing treatment. *Heart.* 2011;97:2078-87.

[30] Furushima H, Chinushi M, et al. Ventricular tachyarrhythmia associated with cardiac sarcoidosis: its mechanisms an outcome. *Clin Cardiol.* 2004;27:217-22.

[31] Sekiguchi M, Numao Y, et al. Clinical and histopathological profile of sarcoidosis of the heart and acute idiopathic myocarditis: concepts through a study employing endomyocardial biopsy. I. Sarcoidosis. *Jpn Circ J.* 1980;44:249-63.

[32] Navaneethan SD, Venkatesh S, et al. Recurrent pleural and pericardial effusions due to sarcoidosis. *PLoS Med.* 2005;2:e63.

[33] Fleming HA. Sarcoid heart disease. *Br Heart J.* 1974;36:54-68.

[34] Yoshida Y, Morimoto S, et al. Incidence of cardiac sarcoidosis in Japanese patients with highdegree atrioventricular block. *Am Heart J.* 1997;134:382–6.

[35] Gozo EG, Cosnow I, et al. The heart in sarcoidosis. *Chest Am Coll Chest Phys.* 1971;60:379–88.

[36] Abeler V. Sarcoidosis of the cardiac conducting system. *Am Heart J.* 1979;97:701–7.

[37] Ton K, Schulman S, et al. Cardiac Sarcoidosis Presenting as Sick Sinus Syndrome and Recurrent Ventricular Tachycardia. *HRS 2014.* 2014. pp. 1-1.

[38] Yazaki Y, Isobe M, et al. Comparison of clinical features and prognosis of cardiac sarcoidosis and idiopathic dilated cardiomyopathy. *Am J Cardiol.* 1998;15:537-40.

[39] Schuller JL, Zipse M, et al. Implantable cardioverter defibrillator therapy in patients with cardiac sarcoidosis. *J Cardiovasc Electrophysiol.* 2012;23:925-9.

[40] Zipse MM, Schuller JL, et al. Atrial Arrhythmias are Common and Arise from Diverse Mechanisms in Patients with Cardiac Sarcoidosis. *Heart Rhythm 2013.* 2013. pp. 1-2.

[41] Viles-Gonzalez JF, Pastori L, et al. Supraventricular arrhythmias in patients with cardiac sarcoidosis prevalence, predictors, and clinical implications. *Chest.* 2013;143:1085-90.

[42] Cain MA, Metzl MD, et al. Cardiac sarcoidosis detected by late gadolinium enhancement and prevalence of atrial arrhythmias. *Am J Cardiol.* 2014;113(9):1556–60.

[43] Winters SL, Cohen M, et al. Sustained ventricular tachycardia associated with sarcoidosis: assessment of the underlying cardiac anatomy and the prospective utility of programmed ventricular stimulation, drug therapy and an implantable antitachycardia device. *JAC.* 1991;18:937-43.

[44] Koplan BA, Soejima K, et al. Refractory ventricular tachycardia secondary to cardiac sarcoid: electrophysiologic characteristics, mapping, and ablation. *Heart Rhythm.* 2006;3:924–9.

[45] Jefic D, Joel B, et al. Role of radiofrequency catheter ablation of ventricular tachycardia in cardiac sarcoidosis: report from a multicenter registry. *Heart Rhythm.* 2009;6:189-95.

[46] Stees CS, Khoo MSC, et al. Ventricular tachycardia storm successfully treated with immunosuppression and catheter ablation in a patient with cardiac sarcoidosis. *J Cardiovasc Electrophysiol.* 2011;22:210-3.

[47] Lubitz SA, Goldbarg SH, et al. Sudden cardiac death in infiltrative cardiomyopathies: sarcoidosis, scleroderma, amyloidosis, hemachromatosis. *Prog Cardiovasc Dis.* 2008;51:58-73.

[48] Hiraga H, Iwai K, et al. Guidelines for diagnosis of cardiac sarcoidosis, study report on diffuse pulmonary diseases. *Tokyo: The Japanese Ministry of Health and Welfare*, 1993;23-24 (in Japanese).

[49] Diagnostic standard and guidelines for sarcoidosis. *Jpn J Sarcoidosis Granulomatous Disorders.* 2007;27:89-102 (in Japanese).

[50] Soejima K, Yada H. The work-up and management of patients with apparent or subclinical cardiac sarcoidosis: with emphasis on the associated heart rhythm abnormalities. *J Cardiovasc Electrophysiol.* 2009;20:578-83.

[51] Ohira H, Tsujino I, et al. Myocardial imaging with 18F-fluoro-2-deoxyglucose positron emission tomography and magnetic resonance imaging in sarcoidosis. *Eur J Nucl Med Mol Imaging.* 2008;35:933-41.
[52] Blankstein R, Osborne M, et al. Cardiac positron emission tomography enhances prognostic assessments of patients with suspected cardiac sarcoidosis. *J Am Coll Cardiol.* 2013;pii: S0735-1097(13)05455-7.
[53] Okumura W, Iwasaki T, et al. Usefulness of fasting 18F-FDG PET in identification of cardiac sarcoidosis. *J Nucl Med.* 2004;45:1989-98.
[54] Ishimaru S, Tsujino I, et al. Focal uptake on 18F-fluoro-2-deoxyglucose positron emission tomography images indicates cardiac involvement of sarcoidosis. *Eur Heart J* 2005;26:1538-43.
[55] Langah R, Spicer K, et al. Effectiveness of prolonged fasting 18f-FDG PET-CT in the detection of cardiac sarcoidosis. *J Nucl Cardiol.* 2009;16:801-10.
[56] Tahara N, Tahara A, et al. Heterogeneous myocardial FDG uptake and the disease activity in cardiac sarcoidosis. *JACC Cardiovasc Imaging.* 2010;3:1219-28.
[57] Yamagishi H, Shirai N, et al. Identification of cardiac sarcoidosis with (13)NNH(3)/(18) F-FDG PET. *J Nucl Med.* 2003;44:1030-36.
[58] Manabe O, Ohira H, et al. Elevated 18F-fluorodoexyglucose uptake in the interventricular septum is associated with atrioventricular block in patients with suspected cardiac involvement sarcoidosis. *Eur J Nucl Med Mol Imaging.* 2013;40:1558-66.
[59] Mc Ardle BA, Birnie DH, et al. Is there an association between clinical presentation and the location and extent of myocardial involvement of cardiac sarcoidosis as assessed by 18F-fluorodoexyglucose positron emission tomography? *Circ Cardiovasc Imaging.* 2013;6:617-26.
[60] Nery PB, Mc Ardle BA, et al. Prevalence of Cardiac Sarcoidosis in Patients Presenting with Monomorphic Ventricular Tachycardia. *Pacing and Clinical Electrophysiology.* 2013;3:364-74.
[61] Schuller JL, Olson MD, et al. Electrocardiographic characteristics in patients with pulmonary sarcoidosis indicating cardiac involvement. *J Cardiovasc Electrophysiol.* 2011;22:1243-8.
[62] Lewin RF, Mor R, et al. Echocardiographic evaluation of patients with systemic sarcoidosis. *Am Heart J.* 1985;110:116-22.
[63] Sekhri V, Sanal S, et al. Cardiac sarcoidosis: a comprehensive review *Arch Med Sci.* 2011;7:546-54.
[64] Suzuki T, Kanda T, et al. Holter monitoring as a noninvasive indicator of cardiac involvement in sarcoidosis. *Chest.* 1994;106:1021-4.

[65] Nery PB, Keren A, et al. Isolated cardiac sarcoidosis: establishing the diagnosis with electroanatomic mapping-guided endomyocardial biopsy. *Can J Cardiol.* 2013;29(1015):e1–3.
[66] Pieroni M, Dello Russo A, et al. High prevalence of myocarditis mimicking arrhythmogenic right ventricular cardiomyopathy differential diagnosis by electroanatomic mapping-guided endomyocardial biopsy. *J Am Coll Cardiol.* 2009 24;53:681-9.
[67] Kato Y, Morimoto S. Analysis of clinical manifestations of cardiac sarcoidosis—a multicentre study: preliminary report, JPN J Sarcoidosis Granulomatous Disord 30 (2010) 73-76 (Japanese with English abstract).
[68] Orii M, Imanishi T, et al. Assessment of cardiac sarcoidosis with advanced imaging modalities. *Biomed Res Int.* 2014;2014:897956.
[69] Greulich S, Deluigi CC, et al. CMR imaging predicts death and other adverse events in suspected cardiac sarcoidosis. *JACC Cardiovasc Imaging.* 2013;6:501-11.
[70] Smedema JP, Snoep G, et al. Evaluation of the accuracy of gadolinium-enhanced cardiovascular magnetic resonance in the diagnosis of cardiac sarcoidosis. *J Am Coll Cardiol.* 2005;45:1683-90.
[71] Patel MR, Cawley PJ, et al. Detection of myocardial damage in patients with sarcoidosis. *Circulation.* 2009;120:1969-77.
[72] Vignaux O, Dhote R, et al. Clinical significance of myocardial magnetic resonance abnormalities in patients with sarcoidosis: a 1-year follow-up study. *Chest.* 2002;122:1895-1901.
[73] Shimada T, Shimada K, et al. Diagnosis of cardiac sarcoidosis and evaluation of the effects of steroid therapy by gadolinium-DTPA-enhanced magnetic resonance imaging. *Am J Med.* 2001;110:520-7.
[74] Yamada S, Kubota K, et al. High accumulation of fluorine-18-fluorodeoxyglucose in turpentine-induced inflammatory tissue. *J Nucl Med.* 1995;36:1301-6.
[75] Mochizuki T, Tsukamoto E, et al. FDG uptake and glucose transporter subtype expressions in experimental tumor and inflammation models. *J Nucl Med.* 2001;42:1551-5.
[76] Mc Ardle BA, Leung E, et al. The role of F(18)-fluorodeoxyglucose positron emission tomography in guiding diagnosis and management in patients with known or suspected cardiac sarcoidosis. *J Nucl Cardiol.* 2013;20:297-306.

[77] Youssef G, Leung E, et al. The use of 18F-FDG PET in the diagnosis of cardiac sarcoidosis: A systematic review and metaanalysis including the Ontario experience. *J Nucl Med.* 2012;53:241-8.

[78] Takeda N, Yokoyama I, et al. Positron emission tomography predicted recovery of complete A-V nodal dysfunction in a patient with cardiac sarcoidosis. *Circulation.* 2002;105:1144-5.

[79] Brudin LH, Valind SO, et al. Fluorine-18 deoxyglucose uptake in sarcoidosis measured with positron emission tomography. *Eur J Nucl Med.* 1994;21:297-305.

[80] Lewis PJ, Salama A. Uptake of fluorine-18-fluorodeoxyglucose in sarcoidosis. *J Nucl Med.* 1994;35:1647-9.

[81] Smedema JP, Reenaers V, et al. Images in cardiology. Cardiac sarcoidosis in a 60 year old woman. *Heart* 2006;92:688.

[82] Koiwa H, Tsujino I, et al. Images in cardiovascular medicine: imaging of cardiac sarcoid lesions using fasting cardiac 18F-fluorodeoxyglucose positron emission tomography: an autopsy case. *Circulation.* 2010;122:535-6.

[83] Bartlett ML, Bacharach SL, et al. Artifactual inhomogeneities in myocardial PET and SPECT scans in normal subjects. *J Nucl Med.* 1995;36:188-95.

[84] Gropler RJ, Siegel BA, et al. Nonuniformity in myocardial accumulation of fluorine-18-fluorodeoxyglucose in normal fasted humans. *J Nucl Med.* 1990;31:1749-56.

[85] Orii M, Hirata K, et al. Early abnormality detected by speckle-tracking echocardiography in a patient with suspected cardiac sarcoidosis. *J Echocardiogr.* 2013;11:69-71.

[86] Ambrosini V, Zompatori M, et al. 18F-FDG PET/CT for the assessment of disease extension and activity in patients with sarcoidosis: results of a preliminary prospective study. *Clin Nucl Med.* 2013;38:e171-7.

[87] Harisankar CN, Mittal BR, et al. Utility of high fat and low carbohydrate diet in suppressing myocardial FDG uptake. *J Nucl Cardiol.* 2011;18:926-36.

[88] Williams G, Kolodny GM. Suppression of myocardial 18F-FDG uptake by preparing patients with a high-fat, low-carbohydrate diet. *AJR.* 2008;190:W151-6.

[89] Tadamura E, Yamamuro M, et al. Images in cardiovascular medicine. Multimodality imaging of cardiac sarcoidosis before and after steroid therapy. *Circulation.* 2006;113:e771-3.

[90] Pandya C, Brunken RC, et al. Detecting cardiac involvement in sarcoidosis: a call for prospective studies of newer imaging techniques. *Eur Respir J.* 2007;29:418-22.

[91] Alavi A, Gupta N, et al. Positron emission tomography imaging in nonmalignant thoracic disorders. *Semin Nucl Med.* 2002;32:293-321.

[92] Chang JM, Lee HJ, et al. False positive and false negative FDG-PET scans in various thoracic diseases. *Korean J Radiol.* 2006;7:57-69.

[93] Lieberman J. Elevation of serum angiotensin-converting-enzyme (ACE) level in sarcoidosis. *Am J Med.* 1975;59:365-72.

[94] Selroos O, Grönhagen-Riska C. Angiotensin converting enzyme. III. Changes in serum level as an indicator of disease activity in untreated sarcoidosis. *Scand J Respir Dis.* 1979;60:328-36.

[95] Rothkrantz-Kos S, van Dieijen-Visser MP, et al. Potential usefulness of inflammatory markers to monitor respiratory functional impairment in sarcoidosis. *Clin Chem.* 2003;49:1510-17.

[96] Shijubo N, Ichimura S, et al. Analysis of several examinations in 516 histologically proven sarcoidosis patients, Jpn. J. *Sarcoidosis Granulomatous Disord.* 27 (2007) 29-35 (Japanese with English abstract).

[97] Ziegenhagen MW, Rothe ME, et al. Bronchoalveolar and serological parameters reflecting the severity of sarcoidosis. *Eur Respir J.* 2003;21:407-13.

[98] Grutters JC, Fellrath JM, et al. Serum soluble interleukin-2 receptor measurement in patient with sarcoidosis, *Chest.* 2003;124:186-95.

[99] Baba Y, Kubo T, et al. Usefulness of high-sensitive cardiac troponin T for evaluating the activity of cardiac sarcoidosis. *Int. Heart J.* 2012;53:287-92.

[100] Yasutake H, Seino Y, M. et al. Detection of cardiac sarcoidosis using cardiac markers and myocardial integrated backscatter. *Int. J. Cardiol.* 2008;102:259-68.

[101] Orii M, Imanishi T et al. Circulating CD14++CD16+ monocyte subsets as a surrogate marker of the therapeutic effect of corticosteroid therapy in patients with cardiac sarcoidosis. *Circ J.* in press.

[102] Hamzeh NY, Wamboldt FS, et al. Management of cardiac sarcoidosis in the United States: a Delphi study. *Chest.* 2012;141:154-62.

[103] DiFilippo FP, Brunken RC. Do implanted pacemaker leads and ICD leads cause metal-related artifact in cardiac PET/CT? *J Nucl Med.* 2005;46:436-43.

[104] Ghafarian P, Aghamiri SM, et al. Is metal artifact reduction mandatory in cardiac PET/CT imaging in the presence of pacemaker and implantable cardioverter defibrillator leads? *Eur J Nucl Med Mol Imaging.* 2011;38:252-62.

[105] Mehta D, Mori N, et al. Primary prevention of sudden cardiac death in silent cardiac sarcoidosis: role of programmed ventricular stimulation. *Circ Arrhythmia Electrophysiol.* 2011;4:43-8.

[106] Aizer A, Stern EH, et al. Usefulness of programmed ventricular stimulation in predicting future arrhythmic events in patients with cardiac sarcoidosis. *Am J Cardiol.* 2005;96:276-82.

[107] Baughman RP, Ohmichi M, et al. Combination therapy for sarcoidosis. *Sarcoidosis Vasc Diffuse Lung Dis.* 2001;18:133-7.

[108] Baughman RP, DrentM, et al. Infliximab therapy in patients with chronic sarcoidosis and pulmonary involvement. *Am J Respir Crit Care Med.* 2006;174:795-802.

[109] Armstrong D, Gonzalez-Stawinski GV, et al. The Two Extremes of Cardiac Sarcoidosis and the Effect of Prednisone Therapy. *Am J Cardiol.* 2015;115:150-153.

[110] Mantini N, Williams Jr B, et al. Cardiac sarcoid: a clinician's review on how to approach the patient with cardiac sarcoid. *Clin Cardiol.* 2012;35:410-15.

[111] Chiu C-Z, Nakatani S, et al. Prevention of left ventricular remodeling by long-term corticosteroid therapy in patients with cardiac sarcoidosis. *Am J Cardiol.* 2005;95:143-6.

[112] Sadek MM, Yung D, et al. Corticosteroid therapy for cardiac sarcoidosis: a systematic review. *Can J Cardiol.* 2013;29:1034-41.

[113] Yodogawa K, Seino Y, et al. Recovery of atrioventricular block following steroid therapy in patients with cardiac sarcoidosis. *J Cardiol.* 2013;62:320-5.

[114] Kato Y, Morimoto S, et al. Efficacy of corticosteroids in sarcoidosis presenting with atrioventricular block. *Sarcoidosis Vasc Diffuse Lung Dis.* 2003;20:133-7.

[115] Betensky BP, Tschabrunn CM, et al. Long-term follow-up of patients with cardiac sarcoidosis and implantable cardioverter-defibrillators. *Heart Rhythm.* 2012;9:884-91.

[116] Bardy GH, Lee KL, et al. Amiodarone or an implantable cardioverter–defibrillator for congestive heart failure. *N Engl J Med.* 2005;352:225-37.

[117] Writing Committee Members, Epstein AE, DiMarco JP, et al. ACC/AHA/HRS 2008 Guidelines for device-based therapy of cardiac rhythm abnormalities: executive summary: a report of the American college of cardiology/american heart association task force on practice guidelines (writing committee to revise the ACC/AHA/NASPE 2002 Guideline update for implantation of cardiac pacemakers and antiarrhythmia devices): developed in collaboration with the American association for thoracic surgery and society of thoracic surgeons. *Circulation.* 2008;117:2820-40.

[118] Birnie DHS W, Bogun F, et al: HRS expert consensus statement on the diagnosis and management of arrhythmias associated with cardiac sarcoidosis. *Heart Rhythm.* 2014;11:1305-23.

[119] Takaya Y, Kusano K, et al. Outcomes in patients with high-degree atrioventricular block as the initial manifestation of cardiac sarcoidosis. *Am J Cardiol.* 2015;115:505-9

[120] Milman N, Andersen CB, et al. Cardiac sarcoidosis and heart transplantation: a report of four consecutive patients. *Sarcoidosis Vasc. Diffuse Lung Dis.* 2008;25:51-9.

[121] Yager JE, Hernandez AF, et al. Recurrence of cardiac sarcoidosis in a heart transplant recipient. *J. Heart Lung Transplant.* 2005;24:1988-90.

[122] Chang TI, Chi NH, et al. Isolated cardiac sarcoidosis in heart transplantation. *Transplant. Proc.* 2012;44:903-6.

[123] Zaidi AR, Zaidi A, et al. Outcome of heart transplantation in patients with sarcoid cardiomyopathy. *J Heart Lung Transpl.* 2007;26:714-7.

In: Sarcoidosis
Editor: Darren Harper
ISBN: 978-1-63482-891-8

Chapter 3

Urological Management of Sarcoidosis: Clinical Manifestations, Diagnostic Methods and Management Strategies

Wei Phin Tan, M.D.[1], Jeffrey C. La Rochelle, M.D., F.A.C.S.[2] and Christopher L. Coogan, M.D., F.A.C.S.[1,*]

[1]Rush University Medical Center, Chicago, Illinois, US
[2]North West Urology Clinic, Portland, Oregon, US

Abstract

Introduction. Sarcoidosis is multi-system disease of unknown cause which occasionally involves the urinary system. We describe the urological manifestations of sarcoidosis and how the disease may affect the management of multiple urological conditions.

Materials and Methods. A systematic search of PubMed® was performed using the keyword "Renal Sarcoidosis" and multiple

* E-mail: christopher_coogan@rush.edu.

urological terms. We only included articles from the English literature in our review.

Results. Sarcoidosis is a disease where non-caseating granulomas form in various organs in the body, particularly the lung whereas genitourinary involvement is clinically scarce. It can also cause a decline in renal function or may present as nephrolithiasis. Recognizing the disease and providing appropriate treatment early in its course may prevent further renal decline.

Conclusions. Sarcoidosis can be a challenging urological disease to diagnose and treat. Urologists should be aware of the urological manifestations of sarcoidosis to avoid misdiagnoses and provide early intervention.

Introduction

Sarcoidosis is a multi-systemic disease that causes non-caseating granulomas to form in various organs, particularly the skin and lungs. Other sites include the liver, eye, spleen and lymph nodes. It may affect any gender and race but has a 3-4 times higher incidence in African American women (36 per 100,000) compared to Caucasians (11 per 100,000) [1]. The lifetime risk of sarcoidosis in African Americans in the US is 2.4% compared with a lifetime risk of 0.85% in Caucasians [2]. The typical age of presentation is between 20 and 40 years of age [3].

Sarcoidosis rarely affects the genitourinary system without involving other organs, primarily the lung [4]. However, it is important that it remains a possible differential diagnosis when treating patient. It frequently presents with respiratory symptoms such as dyspnea, cough and chest pain. Generalize symptoms such as fever, malaise, weight loss and fatigue are common [5].

One of the most common urological manifestations of sarcoidosis is nephrolithiasis and nephrocalcinosis due to disorders related to calcium metabolism.

Infrequently, it can also mimic serious urologic conditions, such as lymphadenopathy in a setting of a renal, bladder or testicular mass which can confound efforts to stage urologic malignancies. Hence, it is empiric that physicians recognize the disease in its early course and provide prompt treatment when necessary. Corticosteroids are the mainstay of therapy.

Materials and Methods

A systematic search of PubMed® was performed using the keyword "Renal Sarcoidosis" and multiple urological terms. We only included articles from the English literature in our review.

Results and Discussion

Kidney

Nephrolithiasis and Nephrocalcinosis

Patients with renal sarcoidosis typically have disorders related to calcium metabolism leading to renal and electrolyte abnormalities. This is due to hyper-absorption of intestinal calcium due to activated macrophages in sarcoid granulomas which express 1α-hydroxylase, which in turn hydrogenizes 25- to 1,25-dihydroxycalcitriol (vitamin D) [6]. In order to achieve homeostasis, the excessive calcium is eliminated in the urine leading to hypercalciuria which is present in 60% of patients with sarcoidosis [7]. This can result in nephrocalcinosis and nephrolithiasis in 10% of patients [8]. In 2.2% of sarcoidosis cases, nephrolithiasis was found to be the presenting feature of the disease [9]. However, only half of these patients were diagnosed with sarcoidosis at the time of presentation. Nearly all these patients were found to have cutaneous lesions and pulmonary involvement on chest x-ray. Hence, a combination of skin lesions, respiratory symptoms and nephrolithiasis should prompt a physician to perform a thorough history and physical exam, particularly on the African-American population [10].

Nephrocalcinosis is less common than nephrolithiasis and only occur in less than 5% of patients with sarcoidosis [8]. Patients may present with polyuria which is caused by hypercalciuria leading to a less responsiveness of antidiuretic hormone [11]. These patients typically have elevated creatinine and occasionally have hematuria or sterile pyuria on urine analysis.

The treatment for hypercalcemia and hypercalciuria in sarcoidosis is mainly corticosteroids. Steroids cause a down regulation of 1α-hydroxylase in macrophages leading to normalization of serum and urinary calcium levels [12]. Ketoconazole has also been shown to be successful in steroid refractive sarcoidosis patients by inhibiting P450 enzymes [13, 14]. Other alternative therapies for hypercalcemia include bisphosphonates and antimalarial drugs such as chrloroquine and hydroxychloroquine [15]. Patients should also reduce their calcium intake to no more than 400mg/day, reduce oxalate intake, eliminate vitamin D supplements and avoid sun exposure.

Medical Renal Disease

Sarcoidosis can also directly affect the kidney by forming granulomas in the tubular interstitium leading to granulomatous interstitial nephritis (GIN). Sarcoid related interstitial nephritis is usually diagnosed on initial presentation and rarely develops among patients with longstanding sarcoidosis [16]. Most patients with GIN presents with elevated creatinine detected on routine screening or as part of their initial sarcoidosis workup.

There is no single test for diagnosing this disease. It is a diagnosis of exclusion and has to be part of the differential diagnosis especially if there is extra renal involvement of sarcoidosis. Renal biopsy is the best test and may occasionally show non-caseating granulomas in the interstitium. A measurement of 24-hour urinary calcium and serum angiotensin-converting enzymes may also provide additional information for the diagnosis of sarcoidosis especially if the disease is only isolated to the renal system. Patients with reduced glomerular filtration rate (GFR) demonstrated to have GIN should receive glucocorticoids. Most patients would typically show some response to corticosteroids but will not revert to normal creatinine levels due to tubular inflammation and fibrosis in the renal parenchyma. Dosages of 1mg/kg per day of glucocorticoids have been demonstrated to be highly effective among patients with GIN.

There is extremely limited data on patients requiring renal transplant as a result of GIN. There are small sample sized retrospective studies demonstrating that recurrence was observed at a median of 13 months after transplantation suggesting that specific clinical and histologic monitoring be routinely performed during the post transplant period for patients with GIN.

Renal Pseudotumors

Sarcoid infiltration of the kidneys can lead to focal lesions involving the kidney. Occasionally, these isolated lesions are difficult to distinguish from primary renal malignancy, particularly if there are no other signs of systemic involvement of sarcoidosis [17-19].

Generalize symptoms such as anorexia, weight loss and fever are common, and patients may also have hematuria which is typically present in patients with a primary renal malignancy. This is further confounded by the presence of retroperitoneal lymphadenopathy or pulmonary changes which can mimic metastatic renal cell cancer.

Pseudotumor typically appears as a solid hypodense mass on CT scan (Figure 1). The renal contour is usually preserved and the lesion may not be apparent on the CT scan until contrast is administered [20, 21]. Ultrasonography is a poor test to diagnose pseudotumors as they may appear hyperechoic, hypoechoic or not visible at all [18, 22].

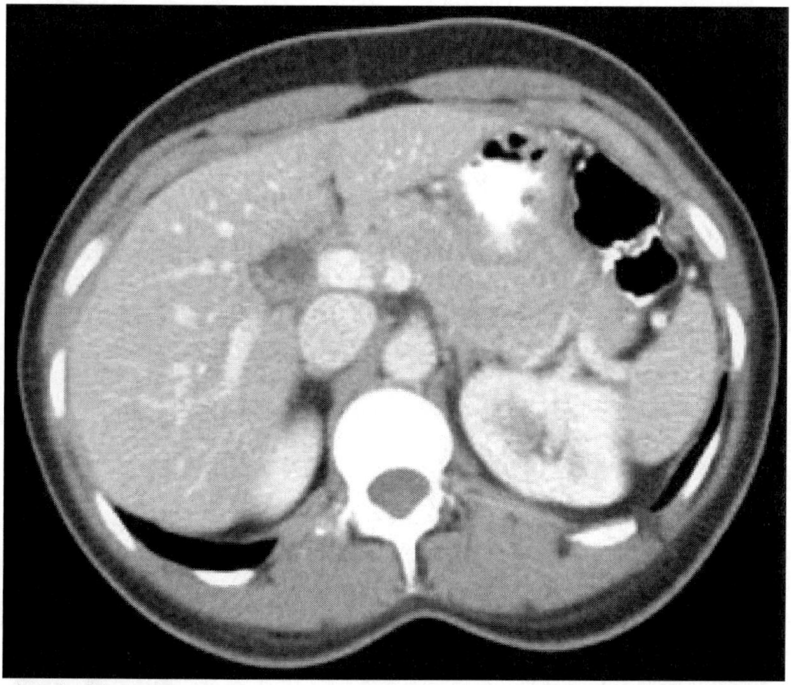

Reprinted with permission.

Figure 1. Sarcoid renal pseudotumor (red arrow).

On Positron Emission Topography (PET), pseudotumor may show an increase in uptake of tracer further complicating the physicians ability to delineate between benign and malignant lesions.

As pseudotumors from sarcoidosis are exceeding rare, a concomitant primary renal malignancy also has to be considered in patients with sarcoidosis. If in doubt, the clinician should consider a percutaneous biopsy if the presenting mass has atypical features. Pseudo tumors from sarcoidosis typically respond well to corticosteroids [23]. In patients with true metastatic renal cell cancer, immunotherapy with interferon and interleukin-2 can worsen the disease process of sarcoidosis [24].

Retroperitoneum and Ureters

Retroperitoneal lymphadenopathy is also a common manifestation of sarcoidosis. Although clinically asymptomatic, severe lymph node enlargement can occasionally lead to ureteral compression leading to hydronephrosis and ultimately renal insufficiency. There have been reports of patient presenting with renal colic subsequently diagnosed to have compression of the ureter from sarcoidosis leading to hydroureter and hydronephrosis [25-27]. Although responsive to corticosteroids, patients who present with retroperitoneal lymphadenopathy from sarcoidosis or retroperitoneal fibrosis typically require urological decompression by double J stent placement or percutaneous nephrostomy tube, and in some cases hemodialysis prior to clinical improvement [28].

Rarely, retroperitoneal fibrosis from sarcoidosis can involve the renal artery causing sarcoid angiitis which may lead to hypertension [29, 30]. This can be diagnosed by performing a biopsy of the renal artery and will typically yield sarcoid angiitis on pathology. Sarcoid angiitis typically respond well to glucocorticoid therapy.

Ureteral obstruction may also occur from renal stones or direct ureteral involvement of sarcoidosis. There have been 2 cases where patients presented with flank pain and were found to have focal narrowing of the proximal ureter [31]. Segmental resection of the ureters in these 2 cases reported non-caseating granulomas on pathology. Hence, it is empiric that patients with a known history of sarcoidosis without any evidence of primary renal tumor undergo a course of corticosteroid prior to any surgical intervention to the ureter.

Bladder and Urethra

Sarcoidosis involvement of the bladder is extremely rare with only 1 isolated report in the literature [32]. However, sarcoidosis can affect the peripheral nervous system in 5% of patients [33]. Neurogenic bladder may arise from involvement of the thoracic spinal cord [34]. These neurological bladder symptoms can present similar to multiple sclerosis and can lead to detrusor sphincter dyssynergia [10].

Another symptom of neuro sarcoidosis is polyuria arising from diabetic insipidus. This occurs through direct hypothalamic involvement leading to central diabetes insipidus or through the hypercalcemia secondary to the production of calcitriol by activated macrophages, leading to nephrogenic diabetes insipidus [35]. Diagnosis is typically made through direct biopsy of the suspected lesion. Corticosteroids are the recommended treatment for neurogenic sarcoidosis. There have also been 2 reported cases of urethral pseudotumors. Both patients were African-American female patients with sarcoidosis and both patients presented with a distal urethral mass which resembled urethral carcinoma. Biopsy however revealed typical sarcoid granulomas and the patients were treated with corticosteroids [36].

External Genitalia

Testis and Epididymis

Epididymal involvement of sarcoidosis is the most common site of sarcoidosis in the genitourinary system [37]. Sarcoidosis may present involving solely the epididymis or it may involve both the testicle and epididymis. The biggest concerns in regards to sarcoidosis of the testis and epididymis are malignancy and infertility. Pseudo tumors in the epididymis can cause obstruction to the vas deferens leading to obstructive azoospermia which may be treated and possibly reversed with corticosteroid treatment [38]. Some authors have recommended pulsed steroid therapy for severe oligospermia. Clinicians should also have a low threshold for sperm banking and repeat lab tests or diagnostic studies as needed [39].

Similar to testicular cancer, sarcoidosis of the testis typically occur between the ages of 20-40 [40]. However, sarcoidosis has a higher predisposition towards the African American population whereas testicular cancer is more common in the Caucasian population. Classic presentation of testicular sarcoidosis is a painless mass in the scrotum. Diagnostic workup includes an ultrasound which commonly shows a hypoechoic or hyperechoic lesion (Figure 2). Management of an intrascrotal mass with a preexisting diagnosis of sarcoidosis can be challenging. Testicular tumor may progress rapidly hence a trial of corticosteroids may be inappropriate as it may result in the tumor growing or metastasizing. Hence, the clinician has to be wary of a pseudo tumor especially if the patient is of African-American heritage, has bilateral lesions and has negative tumor markers. A frozen section or a partial orchiectomy after delivering the testicle through an inguinal incision may decrease the chances of misdiagnosis. The other school of thought is that performing anything less than a radical orchiectomy may outweigh the benefits of a testis sparing approach. There have also been reports of patients with sarcoidosis presenting with mildly increased α-fetoprotein levels which has been theorized to be due to possible sarcoid activity in the liver [41].

Similar to primary renal cancer, it can be difficult to stage testicular carcinoma in the setting of sarcoidosis.

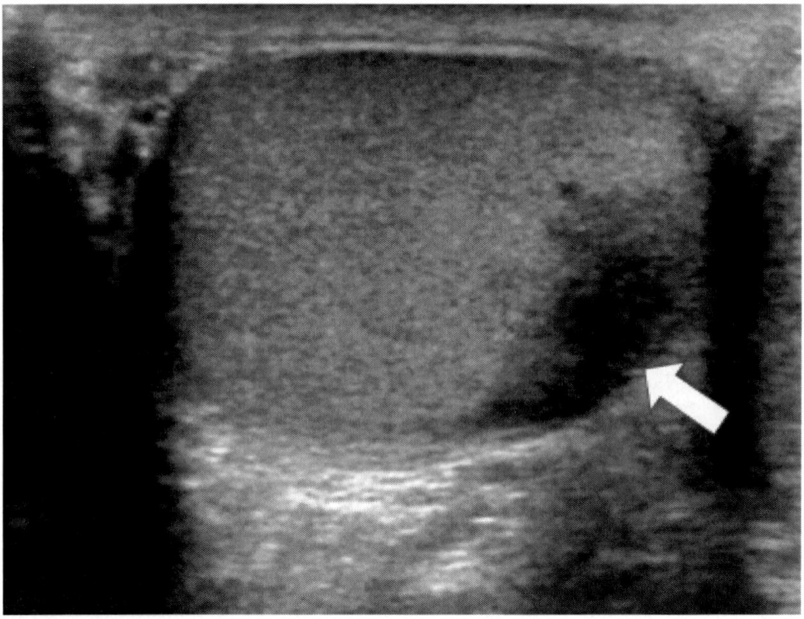

Reprinted with permission.

Figure 2. Scrotal ultrasound showing ill-defined, irregular, hypoechoic lesion at the inferior portion of the right testis (arrow).

Mediastinal lymphadenopathy may be related to sarcoidosis instead of metastatic disease. A biopsy of the mediastinal lymphadenopathy should be performed in patients with sarcoidosis who are diagnosed with testicular cancer. Unfortunately, PET scan is unable to differentiate sarcoidosis and malignancy in the mediastinum [14]. A review of simultaneous testicular cancer and sarcoidosis have demonstrated that sarcoidosis was diagnosed on follow-up imaging of testicular cancer, possibly suggesting that sarcoidosis might arise from a reaction of testicular malignancy [42].

Conclusion

Genitourinary sarcoidosis is uncommon, occurring in less than 0.3% of patients with sarcoidosis. However, because sarcoidosis can happen in any organ and is typically benign and self-limiting, it is empiric that sarcoidosis be considered in the differential diagnosis to begin appropriate treatment. Sarcoidosis can also confound the staging of various urological malignancies and physicians have to know its presentation as not to misdiagnose and provide unnecessary chemo or radiation therapy in the setting of sarcoidosis. Corticosteroid is the mainstay treatment of sarcoidosis and should be started as soon as possible once a patient is diagnosed with sarcoidosis.

References

[1] Rybicki B. A., Major M., Popovich J. et al: Racial differences in sarcoidosis incidence: a 5-year study in a health maintenance organization. *Am. J. Epidemiol.,* 1997; 145: 234.

[2] Rybicki B. A., Major M., Popovich J. Jr., Maliarik M. J., Iannuzzi M. C. Racial differences in sarcoidosis incidence: a 5-year study in a health maintenance organization. *Am. J. Epidemiol.*, 1997; 145(3):234.

[3] Judson M. A., Boan A. D., Lackland D. T. The clinical course of sarcoidosis: presentation, diagnosis, and treatment in a large white and black cohort in the United States. *Sarcoidosis Vasc. Diffuse Lung Dis.,* 2012 Oct.; 29(2):119-27.

[4] Rizzato G., Palmieri G., Agrati A. M., Zanussi C. The organ-specific extrapulmonary presentation of sarcoidosis: a frequent occurrence but a challenge to an early diagnosis. A 3-year-long prospective observational study. *Respiration,* 2005; 72(1):3.

[5] Sharma O. P. Fatigue and sarcoidosis. *Eur. Respir. J.,* 19991 13(4):713.

[6] Bergner R., Hoffmann M., Waldherr R. et al: Frequency of kidney disease in chronic sarcoidosis. *Vasc. Diffuse Lung Dis.,* 2003; 20: 126.

[7] Lebacq E., Verhagen H. and Desmet V.: Renal involvement in sarcoidosis. *Postgrad. Med. J.*, 1970; 46: 526.

[8] Muther R. S., McCarron D. A. and Bennett W. M.: Renal manifestations of sarcoidosis. *Arch. Intern. Med.,* 1981; 141: 643.

[9] Rizzato G., Fraioli P., Montemurro L. Nephrolithiasis as a presenting feature of chronic sarcoidosis. *Thorax*, 1995; 50(5):555.

[10] La Rochelle J. C., Coogan C. L. Urological manifestations of sarcoidosis. *J. Urol.,* 2012 Jan.; 187(1):18-24. doi: 10.1016/ j.juro.2011.09.057.

[11] Procino G., Mastrofrancesco L., Tamma G., Lasorsa D. R., Ranieri M., Stringini G., Emma F., Svelto M., Valenti G. Calcium-sensing receptor and aquaporin 2 interplay in hypercalciuria-associated renal concentrating defect in humans. An in vivo and in vitro study. *PLoS One,* 2012; 7(3):e33145. Epub. 2012 Mar. 5.

[12] Hannedouche T., Grateau G., Noël L. H. et al: Renal granulomatous sarcoidosis; report of six cases. *Nephrol. Dial. Transplant.*, 1990; 5: 18.

[13] Conron M., Beynon H. L. Ketoconazole for the treatment of refractory hypercalcemic sarcoidosis. *Sarcoidosis Vasc. Diffuse Lung Dis.,* 2000; 17(3):277.

[14] Barré P. E., Gascon-Barré M., Meakins J. L., Goltzman D. Hydroxychloroquine treatment of hypercalcemia in a patient with sarcoidosis undergoing hemodialysis. *Am. J. Med.*, 1987; 82(6):1259.

[15] O'Leary T. J., Jones G., Yip A., Lohnes D., Cohanim M., Yendt E. R. The effects of chloroquine on serum 1,25-dihydroxyvitamin D and calcium metabolism in sarcoidosis. *N. Engl. J. Med.*, 1986; 315(12):727.

[16] Mahévas M., Lescure F. X., Boffa J. J., Delastour V., Belenfant X., Chapelon C., Cordonnier C., Makdassi R., Piette J. C., Naccache J. M., Cadranel J., Duhaut P., Choukroun G., Ducroix J. P., Valeyre D. Renal sarcoidosis: clinical, laboratory, and histologic presentation and outcome in 47 patients. *Medicine (Baltimore),* 2009; 88(2):98.

[17] Heldmann M., Behm W., Reddy M. P. et al: Pseudotumoral renal sarcoid: MRI, PET, and MDCT appearance with pathologic correlation. *AJR Am. J. Roentgenol.*, 2005; 185: 697.

[18] Rohatgi P. K., Liao T. E. and Borts F. T.: Pseudotumor of left kidney due to sarcoidosis. *Urology,* 1990; 35: 271.

[19] Yamauchi J., Ubara Y., Suwabe T. et al: Long-term preserved renal function of a patient with mass forming granulomatous interstitial nephritis by biopsy-based steroid therapy. *Clin. Exp. Nephrol.*, 2010; 14: 625.

[20] Koyama T., Ueda H., Togashi K. et al: Radiologic manifestations of sarcoidosis in various organs. *Radiographics,* 2004; 24: 87.

[21] Heldmann M., Behm W., Reddy M. P. et al: Pseudotumoral renal sarcoid: MRI, PET, and MDCT appearance with pathologic correlation. *AJR Am. J. Roentgenol.*, 2005; 185: 697.

[22] Lockhart M. E., Smith J. K., Kenney P. J. et al: Pseudotumorous renal involvement of sarcoidosis. *J. Urol.,* 2001; 165: 895.

[23] Rohatgi P. K., Liao T. E. and Borts F. T.: Pseudotumor of left kidney due to sarcoidosis. *Urology,* 1990; 35:271.

[24] Abdi E. A., Nguyen G. K. and Ludwig R. N.: Pulmonary sarcoidosis following interferon therapy for advanced renal cell carcinoma. *Cancer,* 1987; 59:896.

[25] Fraioli P., Montemurro L. and Castrignano L.: Retroperitoneal involvement in sarcoidosis. *Sarcoidosis,* 1990; 7: 101.

[26] Miyazaki E., Tsuda T., Mochizuki A. et al: Sarcoidosis presenting as bilateral hydronephrosis. *Intern. Med.*, 1996; 35: 579.

[27] Schoenfeld R. H., Belville W. D. and Buck A. S.: Unilateral ureteral obstruction secondary to sarcoidosis. *Urology*, 1985; 25: 57

[28] Fraioli P., Montemurro L., Castrignano L., Rizzato G. Retroperitoneal involvement in sarcoidosis. *Sarcoidosis*, 1990; 7(2):101.

[29] Gross K. R., Malleson P. N., Culham G., Lirenman D. S., McCormick A. Q., Petty R. E. Vasculopathy with renal artery stenosis in a child with sarcoidosis. *J. Pediatr.*, 1986; 108(5 Pt 1):724.

[30] Godin M., Fillastre J. P. and Ducastelle T.: Retroperitoneal fibrosis, renal arterial involvement, and unilateral focal glomerulosclerosis. *Arch. Intern. Med.*, 1980; 140: 1240.

[31] Mariano R. T. and Sussman S. K.: Sarcoidosis of the ureter. *AJR Am. J. Roentgenol.*, 1998; 171: 1431.

[32] Tammela T., Kallioinen M. and Kontturi M.: Sarcoidosis of the bladder: a case report and literature review. *J. Urol.,* 1989; 141: 608.

[33] Burns T. M. Neurosarcoidosis. *Arch. Neurol.*, 2003; 60(8):1166.

[34] Kim I. Y., Elliott D. S. and Husmann D. A.: An unusual presenting symptom of sarcoidosis: neurogenic bladder dysfunction. *J. Urol.*, 2001; 165: 903.

[35] Stuart C. A., Neelon F. A., Lebovitz H. E. Disordered control of thirst in hypothalamic-pituitary sarcoidosis. *N. Engl. J. Med.,* 1980; 303(19): 1078.

[36] Ho K. L. and Hayden M. T.: Sarcoidosis of urethra simulating carcinoma. *Urology,* 1979; 13: 197.

[37] Kodama K., Hasegawa T., Egawa M., et al. Bilateral epididymal sarcoidosis presenting without radiographic evidence of intrathoracic lesion: review of sarcoidosis involving the male reproductive tract. *Int. J. Urol.,* 2004; 11:345-348.
[38] Wong J. A., Grantmyre J. Sarcoid of the testis. *Can. J. Urol.,* 2006; 13: 3201-3203.
[39] Rao P. K., Sabenegh E. S. Genitourinary Sarcoidosis. *Rev. Urol.,* 2009; 11(2):108-113.
[40] Singer A. J., Gavrell G. J., Leidich R. B., Quinn A. D. Genitourinary involvement of systemic sarcoidosis confined to testicle. *Urology,* 1990; 35:442-444.
[41] Sieber P. R. and Duggan F. E.: Sarcoidosis and testicular tumors. *Urology,* 1988; 31: 140.
[42] Tjan-Heijnen V. C., Vlasveld L. T., Pernet F. P., et al. Coincidence of seminoma and sarcoidosis: a myth or fact? *Ann. Oncol.,* 1998; 9:321-325.
[43] Goldsmith S., Harris M., Scherer K., Al-Quran S., Vorhis E. Sarcoidosis manifesting as a psudotumorous renal mass. *Radiology case*, 2013 May; 7(5):23-34.
[44] Kim Y. B., Chung Y. G., Kim S. J., et al. Extensive Systemic Sarcoidosis with Testicular Involvement Mimicking Metastatic Testicular Cancer. *Korean Journal of Urology*, 2011;52(4):295-297. doi:10.4111/kju.2011.52.4.295.

In: Sarcoidosis
Editor: Darren Harper

ISBN: 978-1-63482-891-8

Chapter 4

Cytodiagnosis of Sarcoidosis: Nature of Asteroid Bodies and a Hypothesis on Its Mode of Formation

Dilip K. Das*[*], *MBBS, MD, PhD, DSc, FRCPath.
Associate Professor,
Department of Pathology, Faculty of Medicine,
Kuwait University, Kuwait

Abstract

Sarcoidosis is a systemic disease of unknown etiology characterized by small well-formed granulomas in one or more organs. This chronic multisystem granulomatous disease is often diagnosed after a finding of hilar and mediastinal adenopathy on a chest radiograph. The diagnosis of sarcoidosis needs a compatible clinical picture, as well as demonstrating noncaseating granulomas (without necrosis) in tissues, while other diseases with these features have to be excluded. In patients with suspected sarcoidosis pathologic specimens for diagnosis of sarcoidosis

[*] Address for Correspondence: Dilip K. Das, MBBS, MD, PhD, DSc, FRCPath. Department of Pathology, Faculty of Medicine, Kuwait University, P.O. Box: 24923, Safat13110, Kuwait. Tel: 00965-2531 9476, Fax: 00965-25338905, E-mail:dilip76@hotmail.com.

can be obtained by conventional bronchoscopy with endobronchial and transbronchial lung biopsy, bronchoalveolar lavage, and recently introduced endoscopic ultrasound-guided techniques (endoscopic ultrasound-guided fine-needle aspiration, EUS-FNA, and endoscopic ultrasound-guided transbronchial needle aspiration, EBUS-TBNA) or surgical procedures such as thoracotomy, thoracoscopy, and mediastinoscopy. The diagnostic tools mostly consist of standard TBNA, EUS-FNA and EBUS-FNA. As in histology, the cytologic features of sarcoidosis consist of granulomatous reaction and numerous multinucleated giant cells containing intracytoplasmic inclusions like asteroid bodies (ABs), Schaumann bodies, and/ or calcium oxalate crystals. The sensitivity of these tools in diagnosing sarcoidosis ranges from 60.9% to 100% (median, 86%); specificity ranges~~d~~ from 93% to 100% (median, 100%) and diagnostic accuracy ranges~~d~~ from 73.1% to 95.8% (median, 86.75%). Asteroid bodies (ABs) are commonly described as star-like, spider-, or umbrella-shaped cytoplasmic inclusions in giant cells of granulomas in sarcoidosis and other type granulomas, both of infectious and non-infectious etiology. The pathophysiologic changes that produce ABs, and the nature and significance of these structures seem to be unclear. As early as 1911, intracellular bodies similar in morphology to asteroids were observed in lung, lymph nodes, liver and spleen of autopsy cases before the general recognition of Boek's sarcoid as a disease entity. In the year 1944, the mode of formation of asteroid bodies in giant cells of sarcoid lesions was described but the histochemical reactions failed to give definite information regarding their causation. It took another 25 years, when in ultrastructural studies, the principal materials forming ABs were reported to be either collagen or microtubules, and suggested to be formed by the epithelioid cells themselves or synthesized by distantly located mesenchymal cells and trapped in between epithelioid cells during fusion of epithelioid cells to form giant cells. We have observed that ABs start forming in mononucleated macrophages/epithelioid cells, which may subsequently fuse to form multinucleated giant cells containing one or more ABs. We suggest that the microtubules/tubulins and cytoplasmic membrane forming asteroid bodies in epithelioid histiocytes and MGCs of pulmonary sarcoid lesions, originate from the ingestion of degenerated cilia of bronchial epithelium, which otherwise play a role in the inflammatory process of sarcoidosis including granuloma formation. This hypothesis is based on light microscopic observation of intracytoplasmic material in epithelioid histiocytes having similar tinctorial character as the degenerated cilia in the transbronchial needle aspiration smears, and also cytomorphological evidence to suggest stepwise development of asteroid body from this material.

Introduction

Sarcoidosis is a systemic disease of unknown etiology characterized by small well-formed granulomas in one or more organs that can cause significant morbidity and even death [1, 2]. The prevalence of sarcoidosis ranges from less than one case to 40 cases per 100 000, with an age adjusted annual incidence rate in US of 10.9 per 100 000 for whites and 35.5 per 100 000 for African Americans [3]. This chronic multisystem granulomatous disease is often diagnosed after a finding of hilar and mediastinal adenopathy on a chest radiograph [4]. In asymptomatic state (stage I with bilateral hilar adenopathy on chest radiograph), a presumptive diagnosis can often be made based on a typical constellation of clinical and radiological findings, however, in symptomatic patients the diagnosis of sarcoidosis requires tissue confirmation of granulomatous inflammation [5]. According to American Thoracic Society/European Respiratory Society/World Association of Sarcoidosis and Other Granulomatous Disorders' statement, the diagnosis of sarcoidosis needs a compatible clinical picture, as well as tissue demonstrating noncaseating granulomas (without necrosis), while other diseases with these features have to be excluded [6]. Patients with sarcoidosis usually seek medical attention for the insidious onset of respiratory or constitutional symptoms such as fever, weight loss, anorexia, and night sweats [7]. In biopsy specimens, the granulomas of sarcoidosis show not only asteroid bodies (ABs) but also a number of other cytoplasmic structures/inclusions, including Schaumann's bodies, calcium oxalate crystals, and Hamazaki-Wesenberg bodies [8]. According to Azar and Lunardelli [9], asteroid bodies are rarely observed in thin sections as star-shaped inclusions because of technical difficulties in obtaining a proper plane of section. AB has also been reported in multinucleated giant cells (MGCs) in FNA smears from sarcoid lesions [7, 10]. The pathophysiologic changes that produce ABs, and the nature and significance of these structures, however, seem to be unclear.

Sites of Involvement and the Diagnostic Tools

Since sarcoidosis is a multisystem disease, it has the potential to involve almost any organ system, and has varied clinical manifestations [7]. Thoracic lymphadenopathy is seen in up to 85% of cases [11]. Besides hilar or mediastinal lymph nodes, sarcoidosis can affect lungs, spleen, parotid and thyroid glands, CNS and many other tissues [5]. Cutaneous manifestations in sarcoidosis alone can have varied morphology, ranging from papules, plaques, nodules, lupus pernio, scar sarcoidosis and, rarely, alopesia, ulcers, hypopigmented patches, and icthyosis, which may precede the systemic disease [7]. In patients with suspected sarcoidosis pathologic specimens for diagnosis of sarcoidosis can be obtained by conventional bronchoscopy with endobronchial and transbronchial lung biopsy, bronchoalveolar lavage, and recently introduced endoscopic ultrasound techniques (endoscopic ultrasound-guided fine-needle aspiration, EUS-FNA, and endoscopic ultrasound-guided transbronchial needle aspiration, EBUS-TBNA) or surgical procedures such as thoracotomy, thoracoscopy, and mediastinoscopy [12]. It is suggested that biopsy specimen should be readily obtained from more readily accessible organ using the least invasive method before the treatment is considered [1]. According to Jamil et al. [13], lymph node echofeatures on endoscopic ultrasound (EUS) and concurrent fine needle aspiration (FNA) are alternatives to highly invasive approaches for etiologic diagnosis of mediastinal lymphadenopathy (MLAD). In stage I and II pulmonary sarcoidosis, cellular contents of induced sputum (IS), bronchial washing (BW) and bronchoalveolar lavage (BAL) have been compared in occasional studies [14]. Invasive procedures such as transbronchial biopsy (TBB) or mediastinoscopy may be necessary for diagnosis of mediastinal disease and both procedures have shown a reasonable accuracy in diagnosing sarcoidosis but are associated with a significant rate of major complications and hospitalization is required for mediastinoscopy; on the other hand, the value of cytological examination by fine needle aspiration (FNA) in the diagnosis of sarcoidosis has been shown in various tissues affected by sarcoidosis [5]. In thirty-two FNABs in 28 patients (17 women and 11 men) with cytodiagnosis or differential diagnosis of sarcoidosis, the anatomic sites included lymph node (n=17), lung (n=5), salivary gland (n=8) and liver (n=2) [15]. In patients with clinical and roentgenographic features of pulmonary sarcoidosis, examination with flexible fiberoptic bronchoscopy followed by transbronchial needle biopsy (TBLB) or transbronchial needle aspiration (TBNA) is usually performed [16, 17]. Since intrathoracic lymphadenopathy is common in sarcoidosis (up to 90% of patients), lymph nodes are a likely target to confirm the diagnosis and EUS-guided FNA is an accurate technique for the mediastinal LNs from esophagus, especially those located subcarinally [1, 18]. Transoesophageal bronchoscopic ultrasound-guided fine-needle aspiration (EUS-B-FNA) is not only an alternative to endobronchial ultrasound-guided transbronchial needle aspiration (EBUS-TBNA), it is often more straightforward than EBUS-TBNA with less coughing, and this may be of practical importance to patients with poor lung function or refractory cough [19].

Cytomorphological Features

As in histology, the cytologic feature of sarcoidosis consists of granulomatous reaction and numerous multinucleated giant cells containing asteroid bodies (ABs) and or calcium oxalate crystals [7, 10, 20, 21]. Recently a case of sarcoidosis was reported by Das et al. [21] in which transbronchial needle aspiration (TBNA) smears (Figure 1A) and transbronclial biopsies revealed noncaseating granulomas; in cytologic preparations, asteroid bodies were present in multinucleated giant cells (Figure 1B), binucleated histiocytes (Figure 1C) and mononucleated epithelioid histiocytes (Figure 1D). Presence of ABs in cells other than multinucleated giant cells (MGCs) was described for the first time in this report [21]. In 22 patients with cytodiagnosis or differential diagnosis of sarcoidosis when reviewed, granolomatous inflammation was present in all aspirates, characterized by tightly aggregated groups of at least 10 histiocytes with ovoid to elongated, often twisted nuclei and moderately abundant amphophilic cytoplasm; the histiocyte shape varied from epithelioid to spindilled and multinucleated giant cells and single epithelioid histiocytes were often present in association with granulomas [15]. Mean lymphocyte counts in induced sputum (IS), bronchial washings (BW) and bronchoalveolar lavage (BAL) from sarcoidosis patients are significantly higher than in control patients [14]. In a study of 44 patients with intrathoracic sarcoidosis, cytological examination of bronchial brushings and biopsy imprints revealed epithelioid and/or giant cells in 47% cases in stage 0 and I, in 70% cases in stage II and in 68% cases in stage III; thus cytology is therefore very useful in patients presenting with clinical and radiological picture compatible with sarcoidosis [22]. In six series of cases published during the past decade (2005-2014) primarily under EUS-guidance, the frequency of sarcoid lesions ranged from 2.7% to 42.3%, with a median of 10.6% (Table 1). [13, 23-27] Lohela et al. [28] performed US-guided FNA on 25 nonpalpable supraclavicular lymph nodes clinically suspicious of sarcoidosis; of these 22 (88%) had cytological diagnosis of granulomatous inflammation suggestive of sarcoidosis; three aspirates yielded reactive hyperplasia and 2 specimens were insufficient; the diagnosis of sarcoidosis was confirmed clinically in all the patients during follow up. Mair et al. [29] reported a case of systemic sarcoidosis involving both parotid glands, diagnosed initially by FNA cytology; specific cytological features included epithelioid cells and multinucleated giant cells, without background necrosis. In three cases of sarcoidosis involving the parotid gland as observed by Pérez-Guillermo et al. [10], the fine needle aspiration smears revealed epithelioid granulomas (EG), and multinucleated giant cells (MGCs); asteroid bodies and oxalate crystals were present in one case each.

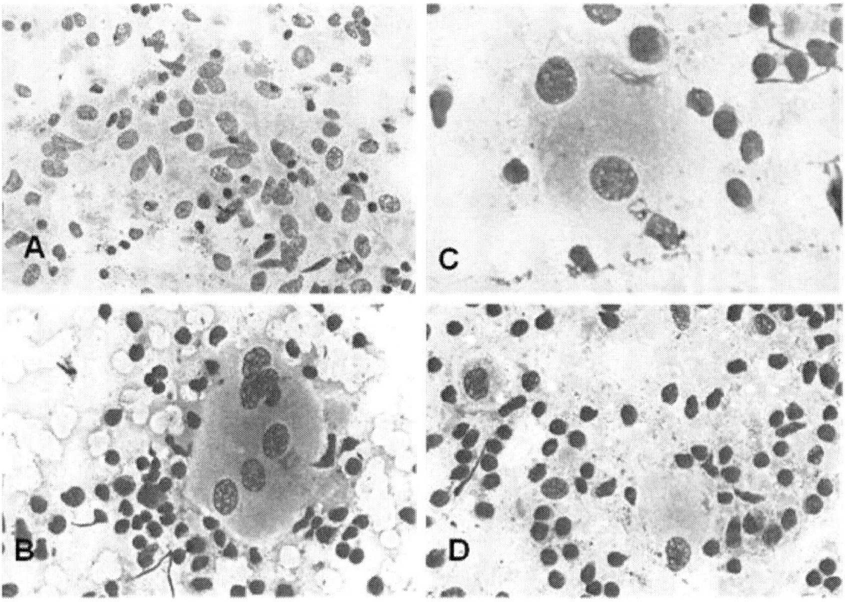

Figure 1. Granulomatous lymphadenitis, with sarcoidosis as a strong possibility. Transbronchial needle aspiration (TBNA) of the enlarged subcarinal lymph nodes in 41-year-old man.
A. A syncytial sheet of epithelioid cells interspersed by a few lymphocytes (MGG x 400).
B. A multinucleated giant cell with two asteroid bodies in close proximity, surrounded by lymphocytes (MGG x original magnification 400).
C. A binucleated histiocyte with a single asteroid body and a few lymphoid cells (MGG x original magnification 400).
D. A mononucleate histiocyte with an asteroid body at the peripheral part of cytoplasm and numerous lymphoid cells (MGG x original magnification 400).

Table 1. Frequency of sarcoidosis in studies based on cytologic specimen

Author and year (Country)	Diagnostic tool	No of cases and sites	No of cases as per tissue diagnosis			
			Malignancy	TB	Sarcoidosis	Others & inadequte
Walsh et al., 2005 (Australia) [23]	EUS-FNA	27 (MLAD)	16	1	3 (11.1%)	7
Khoo et al., 2006 (Singapore) [24]	TBNA & EUS-FNA	20 (MLAD)	15	1	2 (10.0%)	2
Barnett et al., 2009 (USA) [25]	Imaging G. FNA*	131 (para-tracheal)	62	-	10 (9.7%)	59
Fritscher-Ravens et al., 2011 (Germany) [26]	EUS-FNA	72 (MLAD)	4	28	30 (42.3%)	10
Manucha et al., 2013 (India) [27]	EUS-FNA	269 (MLAD)	29†	76 & 123‡	7 (2.7%)	34
Jamil et al., 2014 (USA) [13]	EUS-FNA	160 (MLAD)	60	-	32 (20.0%)	68

*Imaging-guided FNA included endoscopic TBNA, CT-guided percutaneous FNA and endoscopic tranesophageal FNA. †Includes 24 malignant5 and 5 cases suspicious of malignancy, ‡ Granulomatous lymphadenitis diagnosed in 206 cases were finally categorized as tuberculosis in 76, sarcoidosis in 7 and not otherwise specified in 123, MLAD= mediastinal lymphadenopathy.

Differential Diagnosis

Apart from sarcoidosis, the differential diagnosis in noncaseating granulomas includes tuberculosis, histoplasmosis and berryliosis, etc., [18]. Even the cytoplasmic inclusions have been observed in rare instances in granulomatous conditions other than sarcoidosis that includes tuberculosis, leprosy, fungal infections, schistosomiasis and lipoid/foreign body granulomatous inflammation [7]. Besides the presenting features, imaging studies can be of help to some extent in differentiating these conditions. In a study of mediastinal lymphadenopathy (MLAD) by chest imaging modalities, the median lymph node (LN) axis in the benign group [20.5 mm (6-76)] was significantly shorter than in metastasis [28 mm (9-82)] and sarcoidosis [27 mm (17-50)] groups ($p<0.05$) [13]. In mediastinal adenopathies investigated by EUS-FNA, tuberculosis nodes were found to be significantly smaller than those in sarcoidosis [26].

In an earlier study by Fritscher-Ravens et al., [18]. cytology demonstrated epithelioid granuloma formation in all cases suggestive of sarcoidosis; besides cell debris and necrosis (caseating necrosis), the other features which were prominent in tuberculosis included presence of Langhans giant cells (+++ vs. -), and granulocytes (+++ vs. +); and mycobacterial culture studies were negative in all the patients cytologically diagnosed as sarcoidosis except one, in whom the final diagnosis was tuberculosis. In a case treated as disseminated histoplasmosis, transbronchial FNAB from paratracheal lymph node showed granulomatous reaction and numerous multinucleated giant cells containing asteroid bodies (occurring long after the organism was eradicated) [20]. According to Butt et al., [30]. who followed up 30 patients showing noncaseating granulomas after diagnosis of cancer (29 with mediastinal lymphadenopathy and 15 with pulmonary infiltrates or nodules) and observed recurrence of cancer in three patients, noncaseating granulomas may also occur in patients with cancer who develop lymphadenopathy or pulmonary nodules during follow up. In view of the aforesaid findings, in suspected cases of sarcoidosis a tissue diagnosis is strongly recommended; biopsy specimen should be obtained to confirm the diagnosis of sarcoidosis and to exclude the malignant disease, tuberculosis and histoplasma infection [1, 14].

Diagnostic Yield and Efficacy of Cytologic Tools

BAL alone with a diagnostic yield of 47% [31], is not is not adequate and accurate method for diagnosis of sarcoidosis. Flexible bronchoscopy with a diagnostic yield of about 65% (40-90%) reported in several case series is the initial procedure of choice, since the procedure is cheap and can be safely performed on outpatient basis [32]. The sensitivity, specificity and diagnostic accuracy of cytodiagnostic tools for mediastinal/hilar lymphadenopathy involved by sarcoid granuloma and pulmonary sarcoidosis have been shown in table 2 [5, 18, 25, 26, 31, 33-39]. The diagnostic tools mostly consisted of standard TBNA, EUS-FNA and EBUS-FNA. The sensitivity of these tools in diagnosing sarcoidosis ranged from 60.9% to 100% (median, 86%); specificity ranged from 93% to 100% (median, 100%) and diagnostic accuracy ranged from 73.1% to 95.8% (median, 86.75%).

Table 2. Efficacy of Cytodiagnostic Tools in Sarcoidosis

Author and Year	Diagnostic tool	No of cases and sites	Diagnostic efficacy in percentages		
			Sensitivity	Specificity	Accuracy
Fritscher-Ravens et al., 2000 [18]	EUS-FNA	19 (MLAD)	94	100	-
Trisolini et al., 2004 [33]	TBNA	32 (Hilar & MLAD)	65.6‡	-	-
Wildi et al., 2004 [5]	EUS-FNA	124 (HIlar LN)	89	96	-
Wong et al., 2007 [34]	EBUS-TBNA	64 (MLAD)	-	-	87.5
Garwood et al., 2007 [31]	EBUS-TBNA	48(Pulmonary)	85	-	-
Michael et al., 2008 [35]	EUS-FNA	21 (MLAD & abd. LN)	-	-	86
Barnett et al., 2009 [25]	*Imaging-guided FNA	131 (para-tracheal LN)	97	100	79
Tremblay et al., 2009 [36]	Standard TBNA	26 (MLAD)	60.9	100	73.1
	EBUS-TBNA	24 (MLAD)	83	100	95.8
von Bartheld et al., 2010 [37]	EUS-FNA	101 (MLAD)	87	-	-
Fritscher-Ravens et al., 2011 [26]	EUS-FNA	71 (MLAD)	100	93	89
Gimeno-Garcia et al., 2014 [38]	22-G SF-EUS-FNA	126 lesions from 120 patients‡	83	100	-
	25-G SF-EUS-FNA		88.8	100	-
Dhooria et al., 2015 [39]	EUS-B-FNA & EBUS-TBNA	11 (MLAD)†	72.7	100	-

*Includes endoscopic TBNA, CT-guided percutaneous FNA and EUS-FNA (endoscopic ultrasound-guided fine needle aspiration).† Sensitivity and specificity was for all types of cases, whereas 2 of 4 sarcoidosis cases could be diagnosed.‡ Patients had diagnoses which included cases suspiciuous of lymphoma, GIST and sarcoidosis. MLAD= mediastinal lymphadenopathy,‡TBNA together with TBLB had a diagnostic yield of 93.7%, Abd.= abdominal, LN= lymph node. EUS-B-FNA= endoscopic ultrasound fine needle aspiration with an endobronchoscope, EBUS-TBNA= endobronchial ultrasound-guided transbronchial needle aspiration, 22-G SF-EUS-FNA= endoscopic ultrasound-guided fine-needle aspiration using a stylet-free 22-G needle, 25-G SF-EUS-FNA= endoscopic ultrasound-guided fine-needle aspiration using a stylet-free 25-G needle.

Combination of diagnostic tools increases efficacy in diagnosis of sarcoidosis. According to Pauli et al. [16], transbronchial needle aspiration biopsies revealed noncaseating granulomas in 66.3% of patients but combined with forceps bronchial biopsy, the positive rate increased to 77.8%. Morales et al. [17] studied 51cases of suspected sarcoidosis; the sensitivity of transbronchial needle biopsy (TBLB), transbronchial needle aspiration (TBNA) and combined TBLB+ TBNA in 30 cases with stage I disease were 60%, 53%, and 83%, respectively; in 21 cases of stage II disease, these figures were 76%, 48%, and 86%, respectively. In a study by Trisolini et al. [33], the combination of the two methods (TBNA and TBLB) was associated with the highest diagnostic yield (93.7% overall sensitivity), and allowed significantly better results over both TBNA alone (65.6%; p=0.011) and TBLB alone (62.5%; p=0.005).

Complications due to Diagnostic Procedures

The diagnostic tools used for sarcoidosis usually have no serious complications. However, in a review of 252 patients undergoing EUS or EBUS of mediastinal/hilar lymph nodes, von Bartheld et al. [40] reported mediastinal abscesses in 5 patients of suspected sarcoidosis after EUS- FNA necessitating surgical treatment in 4 patients.

Pathogenesis of Sarcoidosis

Sarcoidosis is a chronic granulomatous disorder characterized by an accumulation of T-lymphocytes, macrophages, and immune-effector cells within affected organs; the current understanding of its pathogenesis is that the following sequential immunological events are involved that finally result in granuloma formation and in some unfortunate courses in fibrosis: (1) exposure to one or several still elusive antigen (s), (2) activation of alveolar macrophages, (3) acquiring T cell immunity against the antigen (s) mediated by antigen processing and presentation by macrophages, (4) generation of specific T-effector cells, (5) induction of granuloma formation, and (6) in chronic sarcoidosis induction of fibrosis [41]. Although an etiological agent for sarcoidosis has not been identified, plausible “sarcoid antigens” include mycobacterial antigens such as mKatG or ESAT-6, antigens from Propionibacterium acne, or even self antigens. It is observed that peptides derived from human proteins such as ATP synthetase or vimentin give rise to self antigens and there is a proliferative response of sarcoid T-cells against these peptides [42].

Nature of Asteroid Bodies

Asteroid bodies (ABs) are cytoplasmic inclusions in giant cells of granulomas in sarcoidosis and other type of granulomas, both of infectious and non-infectious etiology, which vary in size from 5 μm to 30 μm and have up to 30 rays forming a star-like, spider-like, or umbrella pattern [7, 43]. Wolbach [44] in 1911 described intracellular bodies in lung, lymph nodes, liver and spleen, similar in morphology to ABs and staining reactions to these asteroids, in five autopsy cases before the general recognition of Boek's sarcoid as a disease entity, and concluded that the bodies were nonspecific, is not a parasitic organism and is a biochemical reaction of the cytoplasm. In a case of sarcoidosis of liver, Ishak [45] observed that the granulomas (noncaseating) were scattered throughout the liver but the characteristic inclusions in giant cells (for example, Schaumann bodies and asteroid bodies) were not seen in all cases and were not pathognomonic. Caca et al. [46] in a case of conjunctival sarcoidosis reported noncaseating granulomas with a prominent component of asteroid bodies. Pearce and Nolan [47] described a case of sarcoidosis of endometrium with many noncaseating granulomas and asteroid bodies. According to Friedman [48], with hematoxylin and eosin the asteroids were pink; phosphotungstic acid hematoxylin stained the asteroids vaguely bluish or sometimes pale orange; asteroids were reddish violet like cytoplasm in Mallory's connective tissue stain indicating that they were negative for collagen; Masson's trichrome stained the asteroids grey (negative for collagen); hematoxylin and van Gieson's stained the asteroids yellow (negative for collagen); in Wilder's reticulum and van Gieson's stain the asteroids were pale pinkish yellow (negative for reticulum), and Weigert's elastic tissue stain demonstrated no elastic tissue in the asteroids and in the rest of the sarcoid lesions. Thus, the histochemical reactions failed to give definite information as to their causation or histological identity. The radiating filaments of ABs, however, were believed to be composed of cytoplasmic processes, which are ultrastructurally spokes made of fibrillar material, radiating from a granular center and the vacuoles between the spokes contain lamellated, lipoidal myelin figures that may be related to formation of Schaumann bodies [49, 50].

Asteroid bodies are an infrequent finding in fine-needle aspirations (FNAs) and although nonspecific, should raise the concern for sarcoidosis, infection, or malignancy [10]. According to Rajasekharan et al. [7], ABs, though not pathognomonic, may aid in the diagnosis of sarcoidosis, which can be confirmed using radiologic and laboratory findings such as negative Gomori's methenamine silver stain for fungi, fire faracco and Ziehl-Neelsen stain for AFB; and no raised angiotensin-converting enzyme (ACE) level (normal range 8-52 IU/L). Jorns and Knoepp [20] described granulomatous reaction with numerous multinucleated giant cells containing asteroid bodies in transbronchial fine-needle aspiration smears of a paratracheal lymph node of a 74-year-old woman with the history of squamous cell carcinoma and disseminated histoplasmosis. Rodriguez and Barrera [51] reported intracytoplasmic asteroid bodies in some giant cells in dermal granulomas of dermal lobomycosis which is a dermal mycosis produced by Loboa loboi and in which the giant cells phagocytose an overwhelming number fungi; under the EM, the AB consisted of bundles of dense, filamentous material, dense bodies and myelin structures resembling the image of ABs in sarcoidosis. Hanke et al. [52], reported giant cell granuloma in skin lesions for which he proposed the term annular elastolytic giant cell granuloma (AEGCG); the histopathology of the lesions showed many multinucleated giant cells (often with prominent asteroid bodies), histiocytes, lymphocytes, scattered epithelioid cells, total lysis of elastic tissue, no necrobiosis, and absence of both mucin and lipid. In sporotrichosis, the asteroid bodies (AB) are extracellular eosinophilic structures, 15-35μ in diameter, and located within abscesses [53]; sporotrichosis ABs must not be confused with the intracellular AB seen in giant cells of granulomatous reactions, which are filamentous and myelin figures that contain lipid. Hematoidin crystals (HC), which are found where extravassated erythrocytes undergo degradation, show a similar star-shape morphology by both light microscopy (LM) and electron microscopy (EM) like ABs) [54]; by LM the HC demonstrate intense, golden-color, fine threads, both intracellularly and extracellularly, in small and large clusters, and in radiating, star-shape patterns ranging in size from 2 to 200 μm and by EM, the HC were composed of a core of dense phospholipid bilayer tubes surrounded by a halo of myelinoid membranes. Brenner et al. [54], postulated that this shape is due to the physiochemical properties of accumulated lipids which originate from superfluous cell membranes created during cell fusion in the case of AB and after cellular (predominantly red cell) breakdown in case of HC.

In 1944, Friedman [48] described the hypothesis of the growth of asteroid body within multinucleated giant cells with illustrations, wherein ABs were found nowhere except within the cytoplasm of the multinucleated giant cells; in most giant cells the cytoplasm showed a few or many punched out clear areas, often with a tiny, pink-staining sphere or coccoid body in the center of each such vacuole but there were larger vacuoles containing larger spheres, some of which had short, sharp pseudopodia or rays protruding from their surfaces; in other cells these rays had become much longer, additional rays appeared, the structure increased in size until it reached the maximum size observed (about 25 μ). As early as 1969, Azar and Lunardelli [9] conceived that the giant cells were a syncytial mass of partly fused or fusing neighbouring epithelioid cells and postulated that the asteroid configuration probably represents a "cast" of slit-like spaces left at the site of confluence of epithelioid cells, and the collagen giving rise to asteroid bodies; it is either synthesized by the epithelioid cells themselves or synthesized by distantly located mesenchymal cells and trapped in between epithelioid cells during the stage of giant cell formation. According to these authors [9], the presence of unit membranes of cytoplasm deep within Langhans type multinucleated giant cells and in relation to arms of asteroid bodies, supports the concept that the giant cells are a syncytial mass of partly fused or fusing neighbouring epithelioid cells. Till now, nobody has refuted this hypothesis. However, collagenous nature of the asteroid body has been challenged by others. According to Cain and Kraus [55], the asteroid bodies in multinucleated giant cells are related to microfilamentous and microtubular structures of the cell. In a subsequent study, Cain and Kraus [56] described the ABs as structures made up of cytoskeleton, predominantly vimentin filaments and smaller amount of microtubules (MTs) and the stellate form of the aggregations is determined by the pre-existing radial arrangement of the element of the cytoplasm. Gadde and Moscovic [57] also feel that AB is definitely a product of the microtubule system and lack collagen; according to them [57], the spokes are massive bundles of MTs rich in tyrosinated alpha-tubulin co-assembled in phosphorylated linkages with yet unidentified microtubule associated proteins (MAPs) and probably microfilament proteins; cores are masses of pericentriolar material including amorphous tubulins, microtubule associated proteins (MAPs), phosphoproteins, and phospholipids; and the cytoplasmic vacuolations around them reflect a collapse and retraction of intermediate filaments (IFs), indicating substantial ongoing MT depolymerization with disruption of MT-IF interactions. Thus, the aforesaid studies, based mostly on ultrastuctural characteristics of ABs, suggest varying nature of these structures. Is it possible that these observations revealing different nature of ABs either represent different substances produced or engulfed by epithelioid histiocytes/MGCs under different environmental conditions?

It is known that microtubules, composed of alpha- and beta-tubulin as well as variable number of microtubule associated proteins, are an integral part of the cytoskeleton of human cells including monocytes and macrophages, where they bind to endotoxin and partly regulate endotoxin induced inflammatory events such as cytokine production [58]. Some recent studies reveal that macrophages not only express virtually all known collagen and collagen related mRNAs, they produce type VIII collagen as well as type VI collagen, which modulates cell-cell and cell-matrix interactions [59]. Therefore, production of microtubules and collagen by macrophages leading to formation of ABs is possible but these findings do not explain the presence of unit membrane of cytoplasm in relation to arms of asteroid bodies, although free cytoplasmic membrane can become a part of MGCs during the fusion of epithelioid histiocytes. In order to explain this phenomenon, we suggest that in pulmonary sarcoidosis, the microtubules/tubulins giving rise to ABs are engulfed by macrophages/epithelioid cells and MGCs. As regards the source of these materials, cilia of the bronchial epithelium seem to be the most likely candidate. Cilia are membranous extensions at the apical part of ciliated epithelial cells, having diameter of 0.3μm and length of 0.6-0.8 μm and the ciliary axoneme consists of a characteristic 9 + 2 array of microtubules surrounded by a cell membrane [60]. This can explain the presence of both microtubules and cell membrane in the ABs.

According to Reichenberger et al. [61], sarcoidosis is characterized by a T-lymphocyte alveolitis with a typically increased T4/T8 ratio. A report by Kriegova et al. [62], provide support for a role of ciliated bronchial cells in pulmonary sarcoidosis; according to these authors [62], CCX CKR is a decoy chemokine receptor that specifically binds to chemokine CCL19, which is upregulated in sarcoidosis and contributes to the development of alveolitis by promoting CD4+ lymphocyte recruitment; further, CCX CKR expression by ciliated bronchial cells from sarcoidosis patients implicate this receptor in the modulation of immune and inflammatory reactions ongoing in the lung and possibly in other organs involved in sarcoidosis. It is also known that there is low frequency of cilia or even squamous metaplasia with a complete loss of cilia in sarcoidosis as revealed in scanning electron microscopic study. [63]. Further, it is observed that presence of either mucus or ciliated cells in BAL is associated with a significant lower T4/T8 ratio (p=0.009) [61]. It is possible that the ciliated epithelium detectable in BAL in sacoidosis represents the damaged ciliated cells and resultant decreased recruitment of T4 cells?

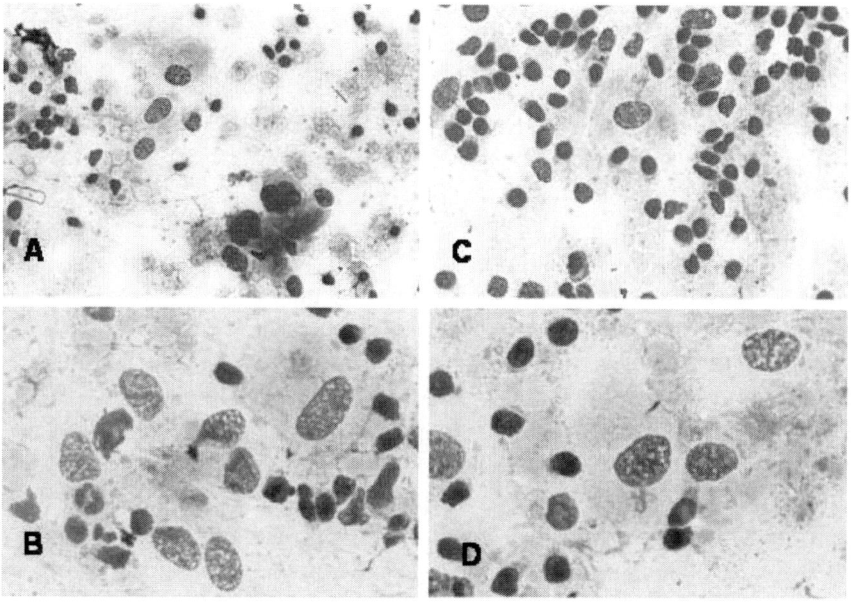

Figure 2. Granulomatous lymphadenitis, with sarcoidosis as a strong possibility in transbronchial needle aspiration (TBNA) of the enlarged subcarinal lymph nodes.
A. An epithelioid histiocyte with magenta colored material in the cytoplasm and a small group of well-preserved ciliated bronchial cells (MGG x 400).
B. Bronchial cells with degenerated cilia and material of similar tinctorial character in the cytoplasm of an epithelioid histiocyte (MGG x 1000).
C. An epithelioid histiocyte with an asteroid body in the stage of organization and magenta colored fibrillar material in another area (MGG x original magnification 400).
D. An almost completely organized asteroid body in an epithelioid histiocyte and a clump of fibrillar material outside which appears to be degenerated cilia (MGG x 1000).

The illness of our patient represented in Figure 1 [21] started with a flu-like illness and six weeks later he presented with persistent cough and difficulty in breathing. The imaging findings revealed air-space disease involving right and left lower lobes and widened mediastinum with bilateral hilar adenopathy. Presence of magenta colored fibrillar material instead of ABs in some epithelioid histiocytes (Figure 2A), prompted us to look for cytomorphologic features, which may throw light on the mode of formation of

ABs. Bronchial cells with partially degenerated cilia, clumps of cilia lying free in the smears and epithelioid histiocytes with intracytoplasmic fibrillar mateial having similar tinctorial character as degenerated cilia (Figure 2B) were observed in this case. ABs in the stage of organization (Figure 2C) and almost well-formed ABs also appeared to be made from these fibrillar material (Figure 2D).

Based on the clinical history and cytologic findings in the present case as well as available knowledge from the literature the following explanation can be offered on the pathogenesis and nature of asteroid bodies. The flu-like or similar illness results in alteration/damage to cilia of the respiratory epithelium. The altered/damaged cilia are engulfed by the macrophages. In order to deal with these engulfed substances effectively, the macrophages seek the help of local helper T-lymphocytes by presenting them with small amount of antigens. Armed with the cytokines secreted by the T-cells, the alveolar macrophages are converted into epithelioid histiocytes and subsequently to typical epithelioid cell granuloma, somewhat similar to granuloma formation in tuberculosis. The similarities between immune responses in sarcoidosis and tuberculosis can be conceived based on the finding that a monoclonal anti-Kviem antibody (IHY-1) reacted on immunoperoxidase staining with epithelioid cells, not only in sarcoid granuloma but also with tuberculous granulomas (although weaker staining) suggesting that the epithelioid cells of granulomas in both sarcoidosis and tuberculosis have a common antigen [64] and what could be this antigen? Heffner suggested that sarcoidosis is an environmental disease caused by noninfectious particulates against a genetic-based dysregulated hyperimmune response [65]. According to Kettritz et al., [66] sarcoidosis shows suppressed immune response to in vivo and in vitro antigen challenges, such as tuberculin, which suggests a state of anergy and a sharp contrast to the accelerated inflammation hypothesis; these authors [66] explain the granuloma formation in sarcoidosis to insufficient suppressive effect on tumor necrosis factor-α, which is central to granuloma formation.

What was the cause of flu-like infection in the case described above by Das et al. [21] is not known, and whether it was a virus, has not been proved. The dynamic events that happen inside the living macrophages in sarcoidosis is not clear. However, based on the morphological observations, it is suggested that the armed macrophages/epithelioid histiocytes try to digest the ingested material consisting of altered/ degenerated cilia with partial covering of cytoplasmic membranes and the latter on their part, try to organize their vibrant microtubules components so as to form asteroid bodies and possibly Schaumann bodies. When these events take place in the lungs and mediastinum, the contribution of degenerated cilia to the formation of ABs can be explained. But how to explain the pathogenesis of asteroid body and/or Schaumann bodies which has been reported in extrathoracic lymph nodes.[7] Some of the macrophages with ingested cilia may be migrating to extrapulmonary sites, being assisted in their movement by the peculiar orientation of tubulins/microtubules in the ABs, and continue to form granulomas there or the granumoma formation start de novo in extrapulmonary sites with ingested material other than cilia, for example collagen, giving rise to asteroid bodies.

References

[1] Newman LS, Rose CS, Maier LA. Sarcoidosis. *N Engl J Med* 1997; 336: 1224-1234.

[2] Peckham DG, Spiteri MA. Sarcoidosis. *Postgrad Med J* 1996; 72: 196-200.

[3] Rybicki BA, Major M, Popovich J Jr, Maliarik MJ, Iannuzzi MC. Racial differences in sarcoidosis incidence: a 5-year study in a health maintenance organization. *Am J Epidemiol* 1997; 145:234-241.

[4] Mishra G, Sahai AV, Penman ID, Williams DB, Judson MA, Lewin DN, Hawes RH, Hoffman BJ. Endoscopic ultrasonography with fine-needle aspiration: an accurate and simple diagnostic modality for sarcoidosis. *Endoscopy* 1999; 31: 377- 382.

[5] Wildi SM, Judson MA, Fraig M, Fickling WE, Schmulewitz N, Varadarajulu S, Roberts SS, Prasad P, Hawes RH, Walace MB, Hoffman BJ. Is endosonography guided fine needle aspiration (EUS-FNA) for sarcoidosis as good as we think? *TThorax* 2004; 59: 794- 799.

[6] Costabel U, Hunninghake GW. ATS/ERS/WASOG statement on sarcoidosis. Sarcoidosis Statement Committee. American Thoracic Society. European Respiratory Society. World Association for Sarcoidosis and Other Granulomatous Disorders. *Eur Respir J.* 1999; 14: 735- 737.

[7] Rajasekharan P, Narurkar S, Patel K, Rajpal A. Asteroid bodies in lymph node aspirate. A case report. *Acta Cytol* 2007; 51: 66-67.

[8] Ma Y, Gal A, Koss MN. The pathology of pulmonary sarcoidosis: Update. *Semin Diagn Pathol* 2007; 24: 150- 161.

[9] Azar HA, Lunardelli C. Collagen nature of asteroid bodies of giant cells in sarcoidosis. *Am J Pathol* 1969; 57: 81-92.

[10] Pérez-Guillermo M, Sola-Pérez J, Espiona Parra FJ. Asteroid bodies and calcium oxalate crystals: Two frequent findings in fine-needle aspirates of parotid sarcoidosis. *Diagn Cytopathol* 1992; 8: 248- 252.

[11] Lynch JP III, Kazerooni EA, Gay SE. Pulmonary sarcoidosis. *Clin Chest Med 1*997; 18: 755-785.

[12] Miliaukas S, Žemaitis M, Sakalauskas R. Sarcoidosis-moving to the new standard of diagnosis? *Medicina (Kaunas)* 2010; 46: 443-446.

[13] Jamil LH, Kashani A, Scimeca D, Ghabril M, Gross SA, Gill KRS, Hasan MK, Woodward TA, Wallace MB, Raimondo M. Can endoscopic ultrasound distinguish between mediastinal benign lymph nodes and those involved by sarcoidosis, lymphoma, or metastasis? *Dig Dis Sci* 2014; 59: 2191-2198.

[14] D'Ippolito R, Foresi A, Chetta A, Casalini A, Castagnaro A, Leone C, Olivieri D. Induced sputum in patients with newly diagnosed sarcoidosis. Comparision with bronchial wash and BAL. *Chest* 1999; 115: 1611-1615.

[15] Tambouret R, Geisinger KR, Powers CN, Khurana KK, Silverman JF, Bardales R, Pitman MB. The clinical application and cost analysis of fine-needle aspiration biopsy in the diagnosis of mass lesions in sarcoidosis. *Chest* 2000; 117: 1004-1011.

[16] Pauli G, Pelletier A, Bohner C, Roeslin N, Warter A, Roegel E. Transbronchial needle aspiration in the diagnosis of sarcoidosis. *Chest* 1984; 84: 482-484.

[17] Morales MCF, Patefield AJ, Strollo PJ, Schenk DA. Flexible transbronchial needle aspiration in the diagnosis of saroidosis. *Chest* 1994; 106; 709-711.

[18] Fritscher-Ravens A, Sriram PVJ, Topalidis T, Hauber HP, Meyer A, Soehendra N, Pforte A. Diagnosing sarcoidosis using endosonography-guided fine-needle aspiration. *Chest* 2000; 118: 928-935.

[19] Medford ARL. EUS-B-FNA for diagnosis of sarcoidosis: A note of caution. *Respiration* 2013; 86:264.

[20] Jorns JM, Knoepp SM. Asteroid bodies in lymph node cytology: Infrequently seen and still mysterious. *Diagn Cytopathol* 2011; 39:35-36.

[21] Das DK, Muqim AA, Sheikh ZA, Al-Kandari M, Junaid TA. Sarcoidosis diagnosed on transbronchial fine needle aspiration smears: a case report with new information on asteroid bodies. *Acta Cytol.* 2010; 54: 225-228.

[22] Leuenberger P, Zellweger JP, Vejdovsky R, Favez G. Histologic and cytologic examination of bronchus and transbronchial lung biopsies at different stages of intrathoracic sarcoidosis. *Schweiz Med Wochenschr* 1981; 111: 98-101.
[23] Walsh PR, Williams DB. Mediastinal adenopathy: finding the answer with endoscopic ultrasound-guided fine-needle aspiration biopsy. *Intern Med J* 2005; 35:392-398.
[24] Khoo K-L, Ho K-Y, Nilsson B, Lim TK. EUS-guided FNA immediately after unrevealing transbronchial needle aspiration in the evaluation of mediastinal lymphadenopathy: a prospective study. *Gastrointest Endosc* 2006; 63: 215-220.
[25] Barnett BP, Sheth S, Ali SZ. Cytopathologic analysis of paratracheal masses: a study of 737 cases with clinicoradiologic correlation. *Acta Cytol* 2009; 53: 672-678.
[26] Fritscher-Ravens A, Ghanbari A, Topalidis T, Pelling M, Kon OM, Patel K, Arlt A, Bhowmik A. Granulomatous mediastinal adenopathy: can endoscopic ultrasound-guided fine-needle aspiration differentiate between tuberculosis and sarcoidosis? *Endoscopy* 2011; 43: 955-961.
[27] Manucha V, Kaur G, Verma K. Endoscopic ultrasound-guided fine needle aspiration (EUS-FNA) of mediastinal lymph nodes: experience from region with a high prevalence of tuberculosis. *Diagn Cytopathol* 2013; 41: 1019-1022.
[28] Lohela P, Tikkakoski T, Strengell L, Mikkola S, Koskinen S, Suramo I. Ultrasound-guided fine-needle aspiration cytology of non-palpable supraclavicular lymph nodes in sarcoidosis. *Acta Radiol* 1996; 37: 896-899.
[29] Mair S, Leiman G, Levinsohn D. Fine needle aspiration cytology of parotid sarcoidosis. *Acta Cytol* 1989; 33: 169-172.
[30] Butt S, Alzebdeh R, Kable TD, Soubani AO. Non-caseating granulomas in patients after the diagnosis of cancer: clinical characteristics and outcome. *Sarcoidosis Vasc Diffuse Lung Dis* 2011; 28: 44-49.
[31] Garwood S, Judson MA, Silvestri G, Hoda R, Fraig M, Doelken P. Endobronchial ultrasound for the diagnosis of pulmonary sarcoidosis. *Chest* 2007; 132: 1298- 1304.
[32] Gilman MJ, Wang KP. Transbronchial lung biopsy in sarcoidosis. An approach to determine the optimal number of biopsies. *Am Rev Respir Dis* 1980; 122: 721-724.
[33] Trisolini R, Lazzari Agli L, Cancellieri A, Poletti V, Candoli P, Paioli D, Alifano M, Tinelli C, Patelli M. Transbronchial needle aspiration

improves the diagnostic yield of bronchoscopy in sarcoidosis. *Sarcoidosis Vasc Diffuse Lung Dis* 2004; 21: 147- 151.

[34] Wong M, Yasufuku K, Nakajima T, Herth FJ, Sekine Y, Shibuya K, et al. Endobronchial ultrasound: new insight for the diagnosis of sarcoidosis. *Eur Respir J* 2007; 29: 1182-1186.

[35] Michael H, Ho S, Pollack B, Gupta M, Gress F. Diagnosis of intra-abdominal and mediastinal sarcoidosis with EUS-guided FNA. *Gastrointest Endosc* 2008; 67: 28-34.

[36] Tremblay A, Stather DR, Maceachern P, Khalil M, Field SK. A randomized controlled trial of standard vs endobronchial ultrasonography-guided transbronchial needle aspiration in patients with suspected sarcoidosis. *Chest* 2009; 136: 340-346.

[37] von Bartheld MB, Veseliç-Charvat M, Rabe KF, Annema JT. Endoscopic ultrasound-guided fine-needle aspiration for the diagnosis of sarcoidosis. *Endoscopy* 2010; 42: 213-217.

[38] Gimeno-Garcia AZ, Elwassief A, Paquin SC, Gariépy G, Sahai AV. Randomized controlled trial comparing stylet-free endoscopic ultrasound-guided fine-needle aspiration with 22-G and 25-G needles. *Dig Endosc* 2014; 26: 467-473.

[39] Dhooria S, Aggarwal AN, Singh N, Gupta D, Behera D, Gupta N, Agarwal R. Endoscopic ultrasound-guided fine-needle aspiration with an endobronchoscope in undiagnosed mediastinal lymphadenopathy: first experience from India. *Lung India* 2015; 32: 6-10.

[40] von Bartheld M, van der Heijden E, Annema J. Mediastinal abscess formation after EUS-guided FNA: are patients with sarcoidosis at increased risk? *Gastrointest Endosc* 2012; 75:1104-1107.

[41] Zissel G, Prasse A, Müller-Quernheim J. Immunologic response of sarcoidosis. *Semin Respir Crit Care Med* 2010; 31:390-403.

[42] Zissel G. Cellular activation in immune response of sarcoidosis. *Semin Respir Crit Care Med* 2014; 35:307-315.

[43] Rosen Y, Vulentin JC, Pertschuk LP, Silverstein E. Sarcoidosis. From the Pathologist's vantage point. *Pathol Annu* 1979; 14: 405- 439.

[44] Wolbach SB. A new type of cell inclusion, not parasitic, associated with disseminated granulomatous lesions. *J Med Res* 1911; 24:243-257.

[45] Ishak KG. Sarcoidosis of the liver and bile ducts. *Mayo Clin Proc* 1998; 73:467-472.

[46] Caça I, Unlü K, Büyükbayram H, Ari S. Conjuctival deposits as the first sign of systemic sarcoidosis in a pediatric patient. *Eur J Ophthalmol* 2006; 16:168-170.

[47] Pearce KF, Nolan TE. Endometrial sarcoidosis as a cause of postmenopausal bleeding: A case report. *J Reprod Med* 1996; 41:878-880.

[48] Friedman M. Sarcoidosis of the spleen: Report of a case with autopsy and a study of intracellular "asteroid bodies." *Am J Pathol* 1944; 20:621-635.

[49] Kirkpatrick CJ, Curry A, Bisset DL. Light- and electron-microscopic studies on multinucleated giant cells in sarcoid granuoma: New aspects of asteroid and Schaumann bodies. *Ultrastructural Pathol* 1988; 12: 581- 597.

[50] Papadimitriou JC, Drachenberg CB. Ultrastructural analysis of asteroid bodies: evidence of membrane lipid layer nature of components. *Ultrastructural Pathol* 1992; 16: 413-421.

[51] Rodriguez G, Barrera GP. The asteroid bodies of lobomycosis. *Mycopathologia* 1996-1997; 136:71-74.

[52] Hanke CW, Bailin PL, Roenigk HH Jr. Annular elastolytic giant cell granuloma. A clinicopathologic study of five cases and a review of similar entities. *Am J Acad Dermatol* 1979; 1:413-421.

[53] Rodriguez G, Sarmiento L. The asteroid bodies of sporotrichosis. *Am J Dermatopathol* 1998; 20:246-249.

[54] Brenner DS, Drachenberg CB, Papadimitriou JC. Structural similarities between hematoidin crystals and asteroid bodies: evidence of lipid composition. *Exp Mol Pathol* 2001; 70:37-42.

[55] Cain H, Kraus B. Asteroid bodies: derivatives of cytosphere. An electron microscopic contribution to the pathology of the cytocentre. *Virchows Arch B Cell Pathol* 1977; 26: 119- 132.

[56] Cain H, Kraus B. Immunofluorescence microscopic demonstration of vimentin filaments in asteroid bodies in sarcoidosis. A comparision with electron microscopic findings. *Virchows Arch B Cell Pathol Incl Mol Pathol* 1983; 42: 213- 226.

[57] Gadde PS, Moscovic EA. Asteroid bodies: products of unusual microtubule dynamics in monocyte derived giant cells. An immunohistochemical study. *Histol Histopathol* 1994; 9: 633- 642.

[58] Allen JN, Liao Z, Moore SA, Wewers MD. Changes in mononuclear phagocyte microtubules after endotoxin stimulation. II. Changes in microtubule composition. *Am J Respir Cell Mol Biol* 1997; 16: 127-132.

[59] Schnoor M, Cullen P, Lorkowski J, Stolle K, Robenek H, Trover D, Rauterberg J, Lorkowski S. Production of type VI collagen by human

macrophages: a new dimension in macrophage functional heterogenesity. *J Immunol* 2008; 180: 5707-5719.

[60] Felix H, Holzmann D. Function and ultrastructure of cilia in primary ciliary dyskinesia. *Schweiz Med Wochenschr* 2000; 130: 699-704.

[61] Reichenberger F, Kleiber B, Baschiera B, Bubendorf L, Brutsche M, Dalquen P, Tam M. Bronchoalveolar lavage quality influences the T4/T8 ratio in sarcoidosis. *Respir Med* 2007; 101: 2025-2030.

[62] Kriegova E, Tsyrulnyk A, Arakelyan A, Mrazek F, Ordeltova M, Petzmann S, Zatloukal J, Kolek V, du Bois RM, Popper H, Petrek M. Expression of CCX CKR in pulmonary sarcoidosis. *Inflamm Res* 2006; 55: 441-445.

[63] Regland B, Cajander S, Wiman LG, Falkmer S. Scanning electron microscopy of the bronchial mucosa in some lung diseases using bronchoscopy specimens. A pilot study including cases of bronchial carcinoma, sarcoidosis, silicosis and tuberculosis. *Scand J Respir Dis* 1976; 57: 171-182.

[64] Ishioka S, Fujihara M, Takaishi M, Yamakido M, Hosoda Y. Anti-Kveim monoclonal antibody. New monoclonal antibody reacting to epithelioid cells in sarcoid granulomas. *Chest* 1990; 98: 1255-1258.

[65] Heffner DK. The cause of sarcoidosis: the centurial enigma solved. *Ann Diagn Pathol* 2007; 11: 142-152.

[66] Kettritz R, Goebel U, Fiebelr A, Schneider W, Luft F. The protean face of sarcoidosis revisited. *Nephrol Dial Transplant* 2006; 21: 2690-2694.

Bibliography

Pulmonary sarcoidosis: a guide for the practicing clinician LCCN: 2013949139 Pulmonary sarcoidosis: a guide for the practicing clinician/Marc A. Judson. Published/Produced: New York: Springer, 2013. Links: Contributor biographical information http://www.loc.gov/catdir/enhancements/fy1404/2013949139-b.html Publisher Description: http://www.loc.gov/catdir/enhancements/fy1404/2013949139-d.html Table of Contents: only http://www.loc.gov/catdir/enhancements/fy1404/2013949139-t.html ISBN: 9781461489269

Sarcoidosis LCCN: 2012540833 Sarcoidosis/[edited by] Donald N. Mitchell ... [et al.]. Published/Created: London: Hodder Arnold, 2012. Description: xvi, 472 p.: ill.; 28 cm. ISBN: 9780340992111 (hbk.) 0340992115 (hbk.) LC classification: RC182.S14 S324 2012 Related names: Mitchell, D. N. Scadding, J. G. Sarcoidosis. Subjects: Sarcoidosis. Sarcoidosis. Notes: Origins in: Sarcoidosis/by J. Guy Scadding. 1967. Includes bibliographical references and index. Dewey class no.: 616.4/29 NLM class no.: 2012 D-947 QZ 140 National bib no.: GBB1B8222 National bib agency no.: 101584482 015946773

Moonlight sonata at the Mayo Clinic LCCN: 2013005858 Moonlight sonata at the Mayo Clinic/Nora Gallagher. Edition: First Edition:. Published/Produced: New York: Alfred A. Knopf, 2013. Description: 207 pages; 21 cm ISBN: 9780307592989 LC classification: RC182.S14 G35 2013 Subjects: Gallagher, Nora,

1949---Health. Sarcoidosis--Patients--Biography. Uveitis--Miscellanea. Dewey class no.: 616.4/29

Harrison's rheumatology LCCN: 2012040104 Harrison's rheumatology/editor, Anthony S. Fauci; associate editor, Carol A. Langford. Edition: 3rd ed. Published/Created: New York: McGraw-Hill Medical, c2013. Description: ix, 358 p.: ill. (some col.); 28 cm. ISBN: 9780071814843 (pbk.: alk. paper) 0071814841 (pbk.: alk. paper) LC classification: RC927 .H376 2013 Variant title: Rheumatology Related titles: Harrison's principles of internal medicine. Related names: Fauci, Anthony S., 1940- Langford, Carol A. Harrison, Tinsley Randolph, 1900-1978. Contents: Introduction to the immune system/Barton F. Haynes, Kelly A. Soderberg, Anthony S. Fauci -- The major histocompatibility complex/Gerald T. Nepom -- Autoimmunity and autoimmune diseases/Betty Diamond, Peter E. Lipsky -- Systemic lupus erythematosus/Bevra Hannahs Hahn -- Antiphospholipid antibody syndrome/Haralampos M. Moutsopoulos, Panayiotis G. Vlachoyiannopoulos -- Rheumatoid arthritis/Ankoor Shah, E. William St. Clair -- Acute rheumatic fever/Jonathan R. Carapetis -- Systemic sclerosis (scleroderma) and related disorders/John Varga -- Sjogren's syndrome/Haralampos M. Moutsopoulos, Athanasios G. Tzioufas -- The spondyloarthritides/Joel D. Taurog -- The vasculitis syndromes/Carol A. Langford, Anthony S. Fauci -- Behcet's syndrome/Haralampos M. Moutsopoulos -- Relapsing polychondritis/Carol A. Langford -- Sarcoidosis/Robert P. Baughman, Elyse E. Lower -- Familial Mediterranean fever and other hereditary recurrent fevers/Daniel L. Kastner -- Amyloidosis/David C. Seldin, Martha Skinner -- Polymyositis, dermatomyositis, and inclusion body myositis/Marinos C. Dalakas -- Approach to articular and musculoskeletal disorders/John J. Cush, Peter E. Lipsky -- Osteoarthritis/David T. Felson -- Gout and other crystal-associated arthropathies/H. Ralph Schumacher, Lan X. Chen -- Infectious arthritis/Lawrence C. Madoff -- Fibromyalgia/Leslie J. Crofford -- Arthritis associated with systemic disease, and other arthritides/Carol A. Langford, Brian F. Mandell -- Periarticular disorders of the extremities/Carol A. Langford,

Bruce C. Gilliland. Subjects: Rheumatology. Rheumatism. Arthritis. Rheumatic Diseases--physiopathology. Arthritis--immunology. Arthritis--physiopathology. Rheumatic Diseases--immunology. Notes: Comprises the rheumatology and immunology chapters from Harrison's principles of internal medicine. 18th ed. 2012. Includes bibliographical references and index. Dewey class no.: 616.7/23 NLM class no.: WE 544

Case studies in neurological pain LCCN: 2012020248 Case studies in neurological pain/Claudia Sommer, Douglas Zochodne. Published/Created: Cambridge: Cambridge University Press, 2012. Description: vii, 142 p.: ill. (some col.); 25 cm. ISBN: 9780521695268 (pbk.) 0521695260 (pbk.) LC classification: RC412 .S66 2012 Related names: Zochodne, Douglas W. Summary: "Among all patients with neurological disorders, pain is probably the most common symptom experienced. Identifying, understanding and treating pain is a responsibility of health care providers in all branches of neurology. This text is about pain in neurological diseases, both 'neuropathic' pain that is recognized in sensory neuron disorders but also other types of pain less commonly considered. These latter disorders include for example, pain in Parkinson's disease, ALS and muscle diseases. The text includes specific chapters on mechanisms of neuropathic pain, updated with new ideas on its pathogenesis, and a Summary: of recent therapeutic guidelines. Most of the text however centers on actual patient encounters at the Neurology clinics of the Universities of Wurzburg and Calgary. This emphasis is to make the vignettes relevant to clinical practitioners but also to introduce researchers and workers in industry to the complex and challenging issues faced during direct patient encounters. Therapeutic failures are common among our vignettes, highlighting the fact that current therapeutic advances remain inadequate-a challenge for researchers to find better approaches"--Provided by publisher. Contents: Machine generated Contents: note: Preface; Part I. The Biology of Neuropathic Pain: 1. Mechanisms of neuropathic pain; Part II. Focal, or Localized Neuropathies: 2. Pain in carpal tunnel syndrome; 3. Pain and cervical radiculopathy; 4. Pain and diabetic lumbosacral plexopathy; 5. Pain and meralgia paraesthetica; 6. Pain and lyme radiculopathy (Borrelia-associated radiculitis); 7. Neuralgic amyotrophy; 8. Painful radiculopathy associated with herpes zoster infection; Part III. Generalized neuropathies or polyneuropathies: 9. Pain and chronic inflammatory demyelinating polyneuropathy; 10. Pain and diabetic polyneuropathy (DPN); 11. Painful idiopathic polyneuropathy; 12. Pain in vasculitic neuropathy; 13. Painful polyneuropathy associated with anti-MAG autoantibodies; 14. Painful polyneuropathy associated with inherited amyloidosis; 15. Small fiber neuropathy in sarcoidosis; 16. Pain and small fiber polyneuropathy in Fabry disease; Part IV. Other Neuromuscular and Neurological Disorders: 17. Pain and proximal myotonic myopathy (DM2); 18. Complex regional pain syndrome; 19. Pain and polymyalgia rheumatica; 20. Phantom pain; Part V. CNS Disorders: 21. Pain in Parkinson's disease; 22. Pain associated with amyotrophic lateral sclerosis (ALS); 23. Pain in Brown-Se;quard syndrome; 24. Pain in syringomyelia; 25. Central pain with thalamic infarct; 26. Pain in multiple sclerosis; Part VI. Headache Disorders: 27. Chronic migraine; 28. Cluster headache; 29. Paroxysmal hemicrania; 30. Trigeminal neuralgia; 31. Headache and acute cerebral ischemia; Part VII. Treatment: 32. Therapeutics in neuropathic pain; Index. Subjects: Neuralgia. Neuralgia. Nervous System Diseases--complications. Notes: Includes bibliographical references and index. Series: Cambridge medicine Dewey class no.: 616.8 NLM class no.: WL 544

The 5-minute pediatric consult LCCN: 2012012664 The 5-minute pediatric consult/editor, M. William Schwartz; associate editors, Louis M. Bell, Jr. ... [et al.]; assistant editor, Charles I. Schwartz. Edition: 6th ed. Published/Created: Philadelphia: Wolters Kluwer/Lippincott Williams & Wilkins, c2012. Description: xxx, 1113 p.: ill.; 28 cm. ISBN: 9781451116564 (hardback: alk. paper) 145111656X (hardback: alk. paper) LC classification: RJ48 .A15 2012 Variant title: Five-minute pediatric consult Related names: Schwartz, M. William, 1935- Summary: "The 5 Minute

Pediatric Consult provides immediate, practical advice on problems seen in infants, children, and adolescents. More than 450 diseases and conditions are covered in the fast-access two-page outline format that makes The 5-Minute Consult Series titles so popular among busy clinicians. Other features include a Chief Complaints section addressing the workup and treatment of 50 signs and symptoms, plus a medication index, syndromes glossary, surgical glossary, laboratory values, and tables all for quick reference saving you time and helping to treat your patients more efficiently.In this sixth Edition:, the 5 Minute Pediatric Consult also offers free 30 day access to the 5minuteconsult Pediatric website -- a clinical decision support tool -- that can be accessed by the health care providers to address questions on-the-go via website or mobile.New Features: New topics for this Edition: include: Amenorrhea, Asberger Syndrome, Dental Trauma, Head banging, Mental Retardation, Narcolepsy, Obsessive Compulsive Disorder, Separation Anxiety and Social Anxiety Free 30 Day Access to the 5minuteconsult Pediatric Website Includes More than 450 diseases and conditions to support your patient care decisions Patient education handouts from AAP to help educate your patients Hundreds of Images from Chung's "Visual Diagnosis and Treatment in Pediatrics" and other reputable sources to provide you with quick visual guidance Immunization schedules and charts at your fingertips to save you time from searching Content is optimized for handheld devices so you have access to the content anytime, anywhere Updates to content made on a regular basis to keep you abreast of the latest content Visit 5minuteconsult.com and click on the "go to pediatric consult tab" to learn more about your free access and begin using today!"-- Provided by publisher. Contents: Abdominal Mass -- Abdominal migraine -- Abdominal pain -- Abnormal bleeding -- Acetaminophen poisoning -- Acne -- Acquired hypothyroidism -- Acute drug withdrawal -- Acute kidney injury -- Acute lymphoblastic leukemia -- Acute myeloid leukemia -- Adenovirus infection -- Alcohol (ethanol) intoxication -- Allergic child -- Alopecia (hair loss) -- Alpha-1-Antitrypsin defficiency -- Altitude illness -- Amblyopia --

Amebiasis -- Amenorrhea -- Anearobic infections -- Anaphylaxis -- Anemia of chronic disease (Anemia of inflammation) -- Anicryptococcal infections -- Ankylosing spondylitis -- Anomalous coronary artery -- Anorexia nervosa -- Anthrax -- Aplastic anemia -- Appendicitis -- Arthritis, Juvenile idiopathic (Rheumatoid) -- Ascaris lumbricoides -- Ascites -- Aspergillosis -- Asplenia/Hyposplenia -- Asthma -- Ataxia -- Atelectasis -- Atopic dermatitis -- Atrial septal defect -- Attention-Deficit/Hyperactivity disorder (ADHD) -- Atypical Mycobacterial infections -- Autism/Pervasive developmental disorder (PDD) Spectrum -- Autoimmune hemolytic anemia -- Avascular (aseptic) necrosis of the femoral head (HIP) -- Babesiosis -- Back pain -- Barotitis -- Bell palsy -- Bezoars -- Biliary Atresia -- Blastomycosis -- Blepharitis -- Bone marrow and stem cell transplant -- Botulism -- Brain abscess -- Brain injury, Traumatic -- Brain tumor -- Branchial cleft malformations -- Breast Abscess -- Breastfeeding -- Breastfeeding Jaundice and breast milk jaundice -- Breath-holding spells -- Bronchiolitis (See also: Respiratory syncytial virus) -- Bronchopulmonary dysplasia (Chronic lung disease of prematurity) -- Bruising -- Bruxism -- Bulimia -- C 1 Esterase inhibitor deficiency -- Campylobacter infections -- Candidiasis -- Carbon monoxide poisoning -- Cardimyopathy -- Cataract -- Cat-scratch disease -- Cavernous Sinus Syndrome -- Cavernous transformation and portal vein obstruction -- Celiac disease -- Cellulitis -- Cerebral palsy -- Cervicitis -- Chancroid -- Chest Pain -- Chickenpox)Varicella, Herpes Zoster) -- Child abuse, Physical -- Chlamydial infections -- Cholelithiasis -- Cholera -- Chronic Diarrhea -- Chronic granulmatous disease -- Chronic hepatitis -- Chronic kidney disease -- Cirrhosis -- Cleft lip and palate -- Clubfoot -- Coarctation of aorta -- Coccidioidomycosis -- Colic -- Coma -- Common variable immunodeficiency -- Complement deficiency -- Concussion -- Congenital hepatic fibrosis -- Congenital hypothyroidism -- Congestive heart failure -- Conjunctivitis -- Constipation -- Contact Dermatitis -- Contraception -- Cor pulmonale -- Costochondritis -- Cough -- Crohn disease -- Croup -- Crying

-- Cryptococcal infections -- Cryptorchidism -- Cryptosporidiosis -- Cushing Syndrome (Adrenal Excess) -- Cutaneous Larva Migrans -- Cyclospora -- Cystic fibrosis -- Cytomegalovirus infection -- 22q11.2 Deletion Syndrome (Digeorge Syndrome) -- Dental/Oral Pain and urgencies -- Dermatomyositis/ Polymyositis -- Developmental disabilities -- Developmental dysplasia of the hip -- Diabetes insipidus -- Diabetes mellitus -- Diabetic ketoacidosis -- Diaper rash -- Diaphragmatic hernia (Congenital) -- Diarrhea -- Diphtheria -- Diskitis -- Disorders of sex development -- Disseminated intravascular coagulation -- Down (Trisomy 21) Syndrome -- Drowning -- Dysfunctional uterine bleeding -- Dysmenorrhea -- Dyspnea -- Dysuria -- Earache -- Edema -- Ehrlichiosis and anaplasmosis -- Encephalitis -- Encopresis -- Endocarditis -- Enuresis -- Endocarditis -- Epiglottitis -- Epstein Barr virus (Infectious Mononucleosis -- Erythema multiforme -- Erythema Nodosum -- Ewing Sarcoma -- Exstrophy of the bladder, cloacal exstrophy, and epispadias -- Failure to thrive -- Feeding disorders -- Fetal alcohol syndrome -- Fever and petechiae -- Fever of unknown cause -- Floppy infant syndrome -- Food allergy -- Food poisoning or foodborne illness -- Fragile X syndrome -- Frostbite -- Functional diarrhea of infancy or toddLer's diarrhea -- Fungal skin infections (Dermatophyte infections, Candidiasis, and Tinea Versicolor) -- Gastritis -- Gastroesophageal reflux -- German measles (third disease, Rubella) -- Giardiasis -- Gingivitis -- Glaucoma-- congenital -- Glomerulonephritis -- Gluecose-6-phosphate dehydrogenase deficiency -- Goiter -- Gonococcal infections -- Graft versus host disease -- Graves disease -- Growth hormone deficiency -- Guillain-Barre syndrome -- Gynecomastia -- Hand, foot, and mouth disease -- Hantavirus -- Head banging -- Headache and migraine -- Heat stroke and related illness -- Hemangiomas and other vascular lesions -- Hematuria -- Hemolysis -- Hemolysis -- Hemolytic disease of the newborn -- Hemolytic uremic syndrome -- Hemophilia -- Hemoptysis -- Henoch-Schonlein purpura -- Hepatic failure -- Hepatomegaly -- Hereditary Angioedema -- Hereditary spherocytosis -- Heroin intoxication -- Herpes simplex virus -- Hiccups --

Hirschsprung disease -- Histiocytosis -- Histoplasmosis -- Hodgkin Lymphoma -- Human immunodeficiency virus infection -- Human papilloma virus -- Hydrocephalus -- Hydronephrosis -- Hyperimmunoglobulinemia E Syndrome -- Hyperinsulinism -- Hyperlipidemia -- Hypertention -- Hypogrammaglobulinemia -- Hypoparathyroidism -- Hypoplastic left heart syndrome -- Hypospadias -- Idiopathic intracranial hypertension (Pseudotumor cerebri) -- Idiopathic Thrombocytopenic purpura -- Immune deficiency -- Immunoglobulin a deficiency -- Imperforate anus -- Impetigo -- In Inappropriate antidiuretic hormone secretion -- Infantile spasms -- Influenza -- Inguinal hernia -- Intestinal obstruction -- Intoeing-tibial torsion -- Intracranial hemorrhage -- Intussusception -- Iron deficiency anemia -- Iron poisoning -- Irritable bowel syndrome -- Jaundice -- Kawasaki disease -- Knee pain, Anterior/Patellofemoral malalignment syndrome -- Lacrimal duct obstruction -- Lactos intolerance -- Lead poisoning -- Learning disabilities -- Luekocytosis -- Lice (Pediculosis) -- Lower GI bleeding -- Lupus erythematosus -- Lyme disease -- Lymphadenopathy -- Malabsorption -- Malaria -- Mammalian bites -- Mastoiditis -- Measles (Rubeola, first disease) -- Meckel diverticulum -- Mediastinal mass -- Megaloblastic anemia -- Meningitis -- Meningococcemia -- Mental retardation -- Mesenteric adenitis -- Metabolic diseases in hypoglycemic newborns -- Metabolic diseases in acidotic newborns -- Metabolic diseases in Hyperammonemic newborns -- Metabolic syndrome -- Methemoglobinemia -- Microcytic anemia -- Milia -- Milk protein intolerance -- Mumps/Parotitis -- Munchausen syndrome by proxy -- Muscular dystrophies -- Myasthenia gravis -- Myocarditis -- Narcolepsy -- Neck masses -- Necrotizing entercolitis -- Neonatal alloimmune thrombocytopenia -- Neonatal apnea -- Neonatal cholestasis -- Nephrotic syndrome -- Neural tube defects -- Neuroblastoma -- Neurofibromatosis -- Neutropenia -- Non-Hodgkin Lymphoma -- Nosebleeds (Epistaxis) -- Obesity -- Obsessive compulsive disorder -- Obstetric brachial plexus (ERB) palsy -- Omphalitis -- Osteogenesis imperfecta --

Osteosarcoma -- Osteomyelitis -- Otitis externa -- Otitis media -- Pallor -- Pancreatic Pseudocyst -- Pancreatitis -- Panhypopituitarism -- Parvovirus B 19 (Erythema Infectiosum, fifth disease) -- Patent ductus arteriosus -- Pelvic inflammatory disease (PID) -- Penile and foreskin problems -- Pericarditis -- Periodic breathing -- Periorbital cellulitis -- Perirectal abscess -- Peritonitis -- Peritonsillar abscess -- Persistent Pulmonary Hypertension of the newborn (PPHN) -- Perthes disease -- Pertussis -- Pharyngitis -- Photosensitivity -- Pinworms -- Plague -- Pleural effusion -- Pneumoystic Jiroveci (Previously known as Pneumocystic Carnii Pneumonis) -- Pneumonia-- Bacterial -- Pneumothorax -- Polyarteritis Nodosa -- Polycystic kidney disease -- Polycystic ovary syndrome -- Polycythemia -- Polyps, intestinal -- Porencephaly cortical dysplasia/neuronal migration disorders-malformations of cortical development -- Portal hypertension -- Posterior urethral valve -- Premature adrenarche -- Premature thelarche -- Premenstrual syndrome (PMS) -- Primary adrenal insufficiency -- Prion diseases (Transmissible spongiform encephalophathies) -- Probiotics -- Prolonged QT interval syndrome -- Protein-Energy malnutrition (Kwashiorkor) -- Proteinuria -- Prune belly syndrome -- Pruritus -- Psittacosis -- Psoriasis -- Pubertal delay -- Pulmonary embolism -- Pulmonary hypertension -- Purpura fulminans -- Pyelonephritis -- Pyloric stenosis -- Rabies -- Rectal prolapse -- Refractive error -- Renal artery stenosis -- Renal tubular acidosis -- Renal venous thrombosis -- Respiratory syncytial virus (RSV) -- Retinoblastoma -- Retropharyngeal abscess -- Reye Syndrome -- Rhabdomyolysis -- Rhabdomyosarcoma -- Rheumatic fever -- Rhinitis, Allergic -- Rickets -- Rickettsial disease -- Rocky Mountain Spotted Fever -- Roseola -- Rotavirus -- Salicylate poisoning (Aspirin) -- Salmonella infections -- Sarcoidosis -- Scabies -- Scarlet fever -- Scleroderma -- Scoliosis (Idiopathic) -- Seborrheic dermatitis -- Seizures-febrile -- Seizures, partial and generalized -- Separation anxiety disorder -- Sepsis -- Septic arthritis -- Serum Sickness -- Severe acute respiratory syndrome (SARS) --

Severe combined immunodeficiency -- Sexual abuse -- Sexual ambiguity -- Sexual precocity -- Short-bowel syndrome -- Short stature -- Sickle cell disease -- Sinusitis -- Sleep apnea--obstructive sleep apnea syndrome -- Slipped capital femoral epiphysis -- Smallpox (Variola virus) -- Snake and insect bites -- Social anxiety disorder -- Sore throat -- Speech delay -- Speech problems -- Spinal muscular atrophy -- Splenomegaly -- Staphylococcal scaled skin syndrome (SSSS) -- Status epilepticus -- Stevens-Johnson syndrome and toxic epidermal necrolysis -- Stomatitis -- Strabismus -- Strep infection: invasive Group A Ç-hemolytic streptococcus -- Stroke -- Stuttering -- Subdural hematoma -- Substance use disorders -- Sudden Infant Death Syndrome (SIDS) -- Suicide -- Superior Mesenteric Artery syndrome -- Superior Mesenteric artery syndrome -- Supraventricular tachycardia -- Sympathomimetic poisoning -- Syncope -- Synovitis--transient -- Syphilis -- Tapeworm -- Teething -- Tendonitis -- Teratoma -- Tenanus -- Tetralogy of Fallot -- Thalassemia -- Thoracic insufficiency syndrome -- Thrombosis -- Tick fever -- Tics -- Toxic alcohols -- Toxic Shock syndrome -- Toxoplasmosis -- Tracheitis -- Tracheoesophageal fistula and esophageal atresia -- Tracheomalacia/laryngomalacia -- Transfusion reaction -- Transient erythroblastopenia of childhood -- Transient Trachypnea of the Newborn (TTN) -- Transposition of the great arteries -- Transverse myelitis -- Trichinosis -- Tuberculosis -- Tuberous sclerosis complex -- Tularemia -- Ulcerative colitis -- Upper gastrointestional bleeding -- Ureteropelvic junction obstruction -- Urethral prolapse -- Urinary tract infection -- Urticaria -- Vaccine adverse events -- Vaginitis -- Vascular brain lesions (Congenial) -- Ventricular septal defect -- Ventricular tachycardia -- Vesicoureteral reflux -- Viral hepatitis -- Volvulus -- Vomiting -- Von Willebrand disease -- Warts -- Weight loss -- West Nile Virus (And other Arbovirus Encephalitis) -- Wheezing -- Wilms tumor -- Wilson disease -- Wiskott-Aldrich syndrome -- Yersinia enterocolitica. Subjects: Pediatrics--Handbooks, manuals, etc. Pediatrics. Pediatrics--Handbooks. Notes: Includes bibliographical references and index. Series: 5-minute consult series 5-minute consult. Dewey class no.: 618.92 NLM class no.: WS 39

Inflammatory diseases of blood vessels LCCN: 2012002558 Inflammatory diseases of blood vessels/edited by Gary S. Hoffman ... [et al.]. Edition: 2nd ed. Published/Created: Chichester, West Sussex: Blackwell Pub., 2012 Description: p.; cm. ISBN: 9781444338225 (hardcover: alk. paper) Related names: Hoffman, Gary S., 1942- Summary: "In recent years, considerable progress has been made in understanding the vasculitic diseases, largely due to the introduction of effective treatments for diseases that were once uniformly fatal, the conduct of structured clinical studies, and advances in immunology and molecular biology. Despite these achievements, the vasculitic diseases continue to be associated with morbidity and mortality from chronic organ damage, relapses, and the side effects of treatment. Investigations into the mechanisms of vascular inflammation may lead to a better comprehension of the pathogenesis of vasculitic diseases and to treatment that is more effective and less toxic. These areas of promising research, together with current knowledge about the vasculitic diseases, are extensively examined in this new Edition:, which is designed to provide a comprehensive overview of the science and clinical consequences of vascular inflammation in health and disease"--Provided by publisher. Contents: Machine generated Contents: note: List of Contributors Preface Section I. Biology of Blood Vessels and Mechanisms of Vascular Inflammation 1. Vascular Development Domenico Ribatti and Enrico Crivellato 2. Vascular Repair Christian Troidl, Kerstin Troidl, Georg Jung, Thomas Schmitz-Rixen and Wolfgang Schaper 3. Leukocyte Trafficking Braedon McDonald and Paul Kubes 4. Dendritic Cells and Vascular Inflammation Cornelia M. Weyand 5. T Cells and Vascular Inflammation Jörg J. Goronzy 6. Autoantibodies and Vascular Inflammation A. Rutgers, J.S.F. Sanders, J.W. Cohen Tervaert, C.G.M. Kallenberg 7. Neutrophils and Vascular Inflammation Matthew David Morgan and Caroline OS Savage 8. Cytokines and Vascular Inflammation Maria C Cid, Marc Corbera-Bellalta, Ester

Planas-Rigol, Ester Lozano, Georgina Espigol-Frigole, Ana Garcia-Martinez, Jose Hernández-Rodriguez, Marta Segarra 9. Oxidative Stress and Vascular Inflammation David G. Harrison 10. Hemostasis and Vascular Inflammation Lawrence Leung and John Morser 11. Animal Models of Vasculitis Masato Nose 12. Arteries, Smooth Muscle Cells, and Genetic Causes of Thoracic Aortic Aneurysms Amy J. Reid and Dianna M. Milewicz 13. Innate Immunity in Atherosclerosis Shuang Chen, Prediman K. Shah and Moshe Arditi 14. Adaptive Immunity in Atherosclerosis Jan Nilsson Section II. Primary Autoimmune Vascular Diseases 15. Historical Perspectives Vasculitis Eric L. Matteson 16. Approach to the Differential Diagnosis of Vasculitis Eamonn S. Molloy and Carol A. Langford 17. Imaging of medium and large vessels (CT/PET/MR) Thorsten Alexander Bley 18. Kawasaki disease Rae S.M. Yeung 19. Henoch-Schonlein Purpura Philip J. Hashkes and Alexandra Villa-Forte 20. Polyarteritis Nodosa Eli M. Miloslavsky and John H. Stone 21. Microscopic polyangiitis Coen Stegeman 22 Granulomatosis with Polyangiitis (Wegener's Granulomatosis) Gary S. Hoffman, Carol A. Langford and Ulrich Specks 23. Churg-Strauss Syndrome (Eosinophilic Granulomatosis with Polyangiitis, EGPA) Christian Pagnoux and Loic Guillevin 24. Giant cell arteritisCornelia M. Weyand and Jörg J. Goronzy 25. Takayasu's arteritis Kathleen Maksimowicz-McKinnon and Gary S. Hoffman 26. Behçet's Syndrome Yusuf Yazici, Ismail Simsek and Hasan Yazici 27. Cogan's Syndrome Rex M. McCallum and E. William St. Clair 28. Idiopathic cryoglobulinemic vasculitides Benjamin Terrier and Patrice Cacoub 29. Primary central nervous system vasculitis Rula A. Hajj-Ali and Leonard H. Calabrese 30. Single organ vasculitis Jose Hernández-Rodriguez and Gary S. Hoffman 31. Primary cutaneous vasculitis Jeffrey P. Callen 32. Buerger's disease (thromboangiitis obliterans) Ahmet Ruchan Akar and M. Serkan Durdu Section III. Secondary Causes of Vasculitis 33. Virus-associated vasculitides Dimitrios Vassilopoulos and Leonard H. Calabrese 34. Drug-induced vasculitis Peter A. Merkel 35. Rheumatoid vasculitis Kimberly P. Liang, Carl Turesson, Larry W. Moreland 36.

Vasculopathy/Vasculitis and progressive systemic sclerosis Nezam Altorok, Omar R. Kahaly and Bashar Kahaleh 37. Vasculitis and Sjögren's syndrome George E. Fragoulis and Haralampos M. Moutsopoulos 38. Vasculitis in systemic lupus erythematosus Ricardo Garcia and Andras Perl 39. Vasculitis in the Idiopathic Inflammatory Myopathies Frederick W. Miller and Chester V. Oddis 40. Vasculitis and relapsing polychondritis Tanaz A. Kermani and Kenneth J. Warrington 41. Systemic Vasculitis in Sarcoidosis Alexandra Villa-Forte and Gary S. Hoffman 42. Vasculitis as a Paraneoplastic Syndrome and Direct Tumour Invasion of Vessels Claire E. Barber and Simon Carette Section IV. Recognizing Risks and Treating Damage from Vasculitis 43. Cholesterol and Modifications of Cholesterol in Rheumatic Disorders Jan Willem Cohen Tervaert 44. Prevention and treatment of medical complications Atul Khasnis and Carol A. Langford 45. Ophthalmic Risks and Complications Associated with the Treatment of Systemic Vasculitis Steven Yeh and James T. Rosenbaum 46. Subglottic Stenosis of Granulomatosis with Polyangiitis (Wegener's Granulomatosis) Rahul Seth and Daniel S. Alam 47. Sino-Nasal Manifestations of Granulomatosis with Polyangiitis (Wegener's Granulomatosis) Daniel S. Alam, Rahul Seth, Raj Sindwani 48. Neurologic Damage of Vasculitis C. David Lin 49. Endstage Renal Disease and Vasculitis Kirsten de Groot and Charles Pusey 50. Cardiothoracic Surgery for Takayasu's Arteritis and Giant Cell ArteritisTurki Albacker and Lars Svensson 51. Peripheral Vascular Surgery for Takayasu's Arteritis and Giant Cell Arteritis Ravi R. Rajani and Vikram S. KashyapIndex. Subjects: Vasculitis. Arteriosclerosis. Immunologic Factors. Vascular Diseases--immunology. Notes: Includes bibliographical references and index. Dewey class no.: 616.1/3 NLM class no.: WG 515

Sarcoidosis: diagnosis, epidemiology and treatment options LCCN: 2011038565 Sarcoidosis: diagnosis, epidemiology and treatment options/Michael R. Connor and Ryan S. Stevens, editors. Published/Created: New York: Nova Biomedical/Nova Science Publishers, c2012.

Description: xi, 166 p.: ill.; 166 cm. ISBN: 9781621007647 (hardcover) LC classification: RC182.S14 S55 2012 Related names: Connor, Michael R. Stevens, Ryan S. Contents: Recent advances in immunogenetics of sarcoidosis: role of human leukocyte antigen --/Ruth López ... [et al.] -- Nodular sarcoidosis/Subramanian Malaisamy, and Ayman O. Soubani -- Pulmonary hypertension associated with sarcoidosis/Tahuanty A. Pena, Ghulam Saydain, and Ayman O. Soubani -- Nuclear medicine imaging in the diagnosis of cardiac sarcoidosis/Gang Cheng ... [et al.] -- Predictors of health status and symptoms impairment in sarcoidosis patients/Branislav S. Gvozdenovic ... [et al.] -- Imaging findings in sarcoidosis/Maria P. Valencia -- Sarcoidosis and fungi: the case for a relation/Marjeta Terčelj, and Ragnar Rylander -- An experimental model of sarcoidosis using kveim tissue/Colin L. Crawford, and Peter Hardwicke. Subjects: Sarcoidosis--diagnosis. Sarcoidosis--epidemiology. Sarcoidosis--therapy. Notes: Includes bibliographical references and index. Series: Human anatomy and physiology Immunology and immune system disorders Dewey class no.: 616.4/29 NLM class no.: QZ 140

Peripheral nerve disorders LCCN: 2014397727 Peripheral nerve disorders/volume editors, Gérard Said and Christian Krarup. Published/Produced: Edinburgh: Elsevier, 2013. Description: xx, 987 pages: illustrations (some color); 27 cm. ISBN: 9780444529022 (cloth) 0444529020 (cloth) LC classification: RC409 .P455 2013 RC332 .H3 v.115 2013 Related names: Said, G. (Gerard), editor. Krarup, Christian, editor. Summary: "Disorders of the peripheral nervous system (PNS) are the cause of prominent neurological symptoms including weakness, sensory loss, pain and autonomic dysfunction associated with deficits, morbidity and mortality. These disorders may be primary hereditary or cryptogenic neurologic disorders confined to the PNS or part of the pathology of both the central nervous system and the PNS. Most PNS disorders are secondary to other system disorders and may be responsive to treatment of the primary disease. Important advances have been obtained in several areas including molecular genetics, biochemistry, immunology, morphology and physiology that have enhanced our understanding of the causes and consequences of damage to peripheral nerve. Understanding of both these groups of PNS diseases has greatly expanded over recent years and has led to important advances of treatment both to protect and to repair damages of peripheral nerve. This volume provides an overview of the state-of-the-art of examination, diagnosis and treatment of these very diverse disorders and will be of interest to both the research and clinical neuroscience and neurology communities"-- Publisher's Description. Contents: Prelude to the peripheral neuropathies -- Microscopic anatomy: normal structure -- Gross anatomy and development of the peripheral nervous system -- Physiology and pathophysiology of myelinated nerve fibers -- Biology of Schwann cells -- Neurophysiological approach to disorders of peripheral nerve -- Testing the autonomic nervous system -- Imaging of the peripheral nervous system -- The nerve biopsy: indications, technical aspects, and contribution -- The cutaneous nerve biopsy: technical aspects, indications, and contribution -- Antibody testing in peripheral nerve disorders -- DNA testing in hereditary neuropathies -- Examination and clinical care of the patient with neuropathy -- How to explore a patient with a chronic axonal polyneuropathy -- Evaluation of a patient with suspected chronic demyelinating polyneuropathy -- Sensory-motor assessment in clinical research trials -- Management of painful neuropathies -- Diagnosis of brachial and lumbosacral plexus lesions -- Compression and entrapment neuropathies -- Facial nerve palsy and hemifacial spasm -- The Guillain-Barré syndrome -- Chronic inflammatory demyelinative polyneuropathy -- Treatment of chronic inflammatory demyelinating polyradiculoneuropathy -- Multifocal motor neuropathy -- Neuropathy and monoclonal gammopathy -- Vasculitic neuropathy -- Sarcoidosis of the peripheral nervous system -- Leprous neuropathy -- HIV peripheral neuropathy -- Human T-cell leukemia virus (HTLV)-associated neuropathy -- Herpes virus infection in the peripheral nervous system -- Lyme neuroborreliosis -- Diabetic neuropathy -- Biology of diabetic neuropathy -- Uremic neuropathy -- Porphyric neuropathy -- Fabry disease -- Transthyretin familial amyloid polyneuropathy -- Hereditary gelsolin amyloidosis -- Malignant cell infiltration in the peripheral nervous system -- Paraneoplastic neuropathy -- Drug-induced neuropathies -- Late radiation injury to peripheral nerves -- Neuromuscular complications of critical illness -- The surgery of peripheral nerves (including tumors) -- Peripheral neuropathy in the elderly -- Dominant Charcot-Marie-Tooth syndrome and cognate disorders -- Recessively transmitted predominantly motor neuropathies -- Early onset (childhood) monogenic neuropathies -- Hereditary sensory and autonomic neuropathies -- Peripheral nerve involvement in hereditary cerebellar and multisystem degenerative disorders -- Giant axonal neuropathy -- Neurofibromatosis type 1 (NF1): diagnosis and management -- Neurofibromatosis type 2 (NF2): diagnosis and management. Subjects: Nerves, Peripheral--Diseases. Peripheral Nervous System Diseases. Notes: Includes bibliographic references and index. Additional formats: Online version: Said, G. (Gerard). Peripheral Nerve Disorders. Elsevier, 2013 9780444633552 (OCoLC)857277776 Series: Handbook of clinical neurology; volume 115, 3rd series Handbook of clinical neurology; 3rd ser., v. 115. Dewey class no.: 616.85/6 NLM class no.: WL 100 H236 v.115 2013 National bib agency no.: 101627322

Thoracic imaging LCCN: 2014001336 Thoracic imaging/SJ Copley, MD, FRCP, FRCR, Consultant Radiologist and Reader in Thoracic Imaging, Imperial College Healthcare Trust, Hammersmith Hospital, London, UK, JP Kanne, MD, FRCP, CRCR, Professor of Thoracic Imaging, Royal Brompton Hospital, London, UK. DM Hansell, MD, Chief of Thoracic Imaging, University of Wisconsin School of Medicine, Madison, WI, USA. Edition: Second Edition:. Published/Produced: Boca Raton: CRC Press, Taylor & Francis Group, [2014] ©2014 Description: viii, 204 pages: illustrations (some color); 25 cm ISBN: 9781482231151 (pbk.: alk. paper) 1482231158 (pbk.: alk. paper) LC classification: RC941 .C777 2014 Related names: Hansell, David M.

Kanne, Jeffrey P. Summary: "Containing 100 challenging clinical cases and illustrated with high-quality images, this book covers a wide range of conditions from common afflictions such as tuberculosis, pulmonary masses, and mediastinal masses, to the more challenging cases such as cystic fibrosis, asbestosis, sarcoidosis, and alveolar cell carcinoma. The book remains an invaluable text for radiologists and imaging professionals in practice and in training, from hospital-based doctors preparing for higher examinations to established physicians looking to continue their professional development"-- Provided by publisher. Subjects: Thoracic Diseases--diagnosis--Case Reports. Thoracic Diseases--diagnosis--Examination Questions. Diagnostic Imaging--Case Reports. Diagnostic Imaging--Examination Questions. Notes: Includes bibliographical references and index. Series Illustrated clinical cases Illustrated clinical cases. Dewey class no.: 617.5/407572 NLM class no.: WF 18.2

Index

B

C

D

E

F

G

H

I

J

K

L

M

N

O

P

Q

T

U

V

W

Y